SKIN DISEASES

INCLUDING THEIR

DEFINITION, SYMPTOMS, DIAGNOSIS, PROGNOSIS
MORBID ANATOMY AND TREATMENT

A MANUAL
for
STUDENTS AND PRACTITIONERS

BY

MALCOLM MORRIS

JOINT LECTURER ON DERMATOLOGY AT ST MARY'S HOSPITAL MEDICAL SCHOOL
AND FORMERLY CLINICAL ASSISTANT, HOSPITAL FOR DISEASES
OF THE SKIN, STAMFORD STREET, BLACKFRIARS

𝔚𝔦𝔱𝔥 𝔍𝔩𝔩𝔲𝔰𝔱𝔯𝔞𝔱𝔦𝔬𝔫𝔰

LONDON
SMITH, ELDER, & CO., 15 WATERLOO PLACE
1879

PREFACE.

In undertaking this little work, my object has been to supplement, not to supplant, existing treatises upon a subject which it is difficult to condense and arrange, and one, therefore, which has proved tedious to the student.

Commenced some months ago, to assist not only the students, but myself also, in the delivery of a course of Lectures at St. Mary's Hospital Medical School, it has by degrees so far exceeded its original limits as to have suggested the second half of its present title; for, while its simplicity will, it is hoped, adapt it to the wants of the student, its conciseness may commend it to the general practitioner.

To Mr. Jonathan Hutchinson and Mr. Waren Tay I am especially indebted for the useful knowledge which I obtained from them whilst acting as Clinical Assistant at the Hospital for Diseases of the Skin, Blackfriars; and to my friend and colleague, Dr. Cheadle, I owe my sincere thanks for kind assistance and for special opportunities of observing many interesting cases.

Moreover, I have not hesitated in the process of compilation to make constant requisition upon numerous authorities on Dermatology, both British and Foreign.

The Anatomy of the Skin in the first chapter, is founded chiefly upon Biesiadecki's article in Stricker's 'Manual,' and Klein and Noble Smith's 'Atlas of Histology.' The plates which have been placed at my disposal by Dr. Klein form but a part of the kindness I have received at his hands, and which I here heartily wish to acknowledge. For the skilful execution of the woodcuts, I think I am justified in speaking in no measured terms of the able work of Mr. Noble Smith.

I must also express my thanks to my friend, Dr. Alfred Sangster, for much valuable assistance.

M. M.

63 MONTAGU SQUARE, HYDE PARK, W.
November 1879.

CONTENTS.

MANUAL

OF

SKIN DISEASES.

CHAPTER I.

ANATOMY AND PHYSIOLOGY.

ANATOMY.

THE skin is the covering of the body which protects the more delicate tissues from injury, and joins the mucous membrane at the various orifices. The surface is not smooth, but consists of elevations, grooves, and depressions. The elevations form in places, such as the palm of the hand and sole of the foot, lines and wrinkles. The smallest elevations are caused by the prominence of the papillæ of the true skin. The grooves correspond to the lines or wrinkles, and lie between them. The depressions or pores of the skin are produced by the openings of the hair follicles, sebaceous and sweat glands.

The skin consists of two parts—

> The Epidermis,
> The Corium, or true skin,

together with more or less subcutaneous connective tissue. Besides these two layers there are certain structures to be described—viz. adipose tissue, sweat glands, sebaceous glands, hair follicles and hairs, muscular tissue, nails, blood vessels, nerves, and lymphatics.

B

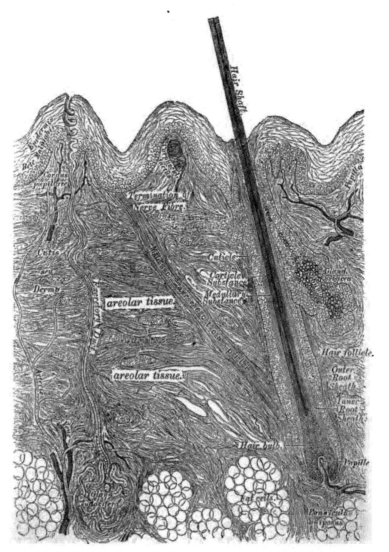

Fig. 1.—GENERAL VIEW OF THE SKIN AND APPENDAGES. (After Heitzmann.)

EPIDERMIS.

The epidermis is composed of four different layers or strata—

1. Rete Malpighii, or rete mucosum.
2. Granular layer.
3. Stratum lucidum.
4. Stratum corneum.

1. *Rete Malpighii.*—This is made up of a stratified pavement epithelium. The cells of the deepest layer are columnar in form, with oval nuclei; above, there are several layers of

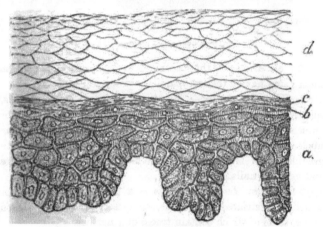

Fig. 2.—THE EPIDERMIS.

a, rete Malpighii; *b*, granular layer; *c*, stratum lucidum; *d*, stratum corneum.
(From Klein and Noble Smith's ' Atlas of Histology.')

polyhedral cells, with more or less spherical nuclei. The most superficial cells and their nuclei are flattened. The polyhedral and the columnar-shaped cells are joined together by fine fibrils, the so-called prickle cells of Max Schultze; these fibres are simply the prolongation of the mass of fibrils that constitutes the chief structure of the cells themselves. Thus the cells are composed of a delicate network, called the intracellular network, and a hyaline interfibrillar substance. Between the cells are the intercellular spaces, which are occupied by a clear semi-albuminous substance, the intercellular cement. In the spaces are seen branched connective-tissue corpuscles, and the termination of nerves extending from the corium.

In dark-coloured skins the deepest cells contain pigment granules. The rete rests upon the true skin, and adapts itself

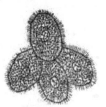

Fig. 3.—THE STRUCTURE OF CELLS. (Klein.)

to the elevations of the papillæ, the prolongations between them being named the interpapillary processes.

2. *Granular Layer.*—This is a layer of flattened cells, spindle-shaped in vertical section, situated on the surface or outer aspect of the rete Malpighii. Each cell contains a clear nucleus, from the ends of which rodlike granules extend. The granular layer is best seen at the mouths of the hair follicles and near the nails.

3. *Stratum Lucidum.*—This is a bright homogeneous or indistinctly striated membrane, composed of closely packed scales, some of which contain traces of a nucleus.

4. *Stratum Corneum.*—This consists of many layers of horny non-nucleated scales. In various parts of the body this layer alters considerably in thickness, being very dense on the palms and soles.

CORIUM.

The corium is composed of connective-tissue elements, in which are embedded various important organs, such as the glands of the skin and their ducts, hairs, blood vessels, and nerves. This connective tissue occurs as a dense felt-work, formed by bundles of fibres, which divide and cross each other repeatedly. Each bundle is formed of fine fibrils that yield gelatine, and are held together by an albuminous fluid cement substance. This substance is also found between the bundles themselves, each of which probably possesses a hyaline sheath as well: acids or boiling cause the bundles to swell up. On account of the difference in density, the corium is said to be divided into two parts; the superficial is known as the papillary body, in which the bundles of connective tissue are very thin, less dense, and hence more transparent. Between the groups of bundles, or trabeculæ, are spaces called lacunæ, which anastomose with one another by means of narrow channels. These lacunæ and channels form the lymph canalicular system, and contain flattened, nucleated, branched connective-tissue corpuscles, the nucleated parts lying more particularly in the lacunæ, while the branched processes extend into the channels. There are certain elevations on the surface of the corium, of various sizes and shapes, called papillæ, between which are processes of the rete Malpighii. The largest are found on the palm of the hand and fingers. Some only contain vascular loops, others also nerve fibres and tactile corpuscles. A thin basement membrane lies between the corium and the rete Malpighii.

SUBCUTANEOUS TISSUE.

In the subcutaneous tissue the bundles of connective tissue are aggregated into larger groups, which do not interlace so markedly as in the corium. Owing to this arrangement of the tissue, it assumes a slightly lamellar-like appearance, but many groups of trabeculæ run obliquely or even vertically, and thus continuous spaces are left between the groups of bundles. Connective-tissue corpuscles line these spaces, and lie on the surface of the trabeculæ in rows of unbranched, flat, endothelial cells. Bright fibrils of elastic tissue, that branch and anastomose to form networks, and vary in thickness, are found also on the surface of the trabeculæ, in close relation to the corpuscles. In some situations subcutaneous tissue contains considerable quantities of fat, and is then called the *panniculus adiposus*; other parts, such as the eyelids, ears, penis, and scrotum, are absolutely destitute of fat. A few migratory connective-tissue cells lie in the spaces of the superficial part of the corium, and also in the subcutaneous tissue, very similar to plasma cells, large, coarsely granular, and exhibiting only slight amœboid movements.

Large blood vessels pass through the subcutaneous tissue, where they give off branches to the corium and the other organs.

ADIPOSE TISSUE.

This tissue is composed of fat cells, which are arranged in groups to form lobules, and these again are aggregated into lobes. The cells are apparently spherical; each contains a fat globule, which occupies the bulk of the cell. The protoplasm of the cell is reduced to a thin wall, in one part of which is seen a more or less compressed nucleus. Between the fat cells there are flattened nucleated connective-tissue cells, and between the lobules there are septa of fibrous tissue, with similar but proportionately larger septa between the lobes. Adipose tissue has characters in common with gland tissue; thus to each lobe and lobule there is an afferent artery and one or more efferent veins, with a network of capillaries encircling the fat cells, either individually or in groups of two or three.

SWEAT GLANDS.

A sweat gland is a tube, composed of a membrana propria and of a lining epithelium, which consists of a single layer of columnar epithelial cells. The gland proper is situated in the subcutaneous tissue, and is formed by the convolution of the deep part of the tube. The duct passes from the gland proper in an oblique and vertical direction through the corium and epidermis to open on the surface. The epidermic portion is called the mouth of the duct; in it there is no membrana propria or special epithelium, and in consequence it is surrounded only by the cells of the epidermis.

The duct is lined at the commencement by a continuation of the rete Malpighii, the cells of which are stratified, but gradually, as the deeper parts are reached, the epidermis is reduced first to two layers of pavement cells and then to a single layer of short columnar cells, which at the lowest portion become elongated.

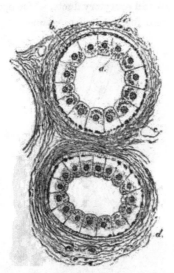

Fig. 4.—TRANSVERSE SECTION OF SWEAT GLAND.
a, epithelium; b, muscular coat cut transversely; c, nucleated membrana propria; d, connective tissue. (Sangster.)

The tube of the gland proper, in some parts of the body, contains a single layer of thin longitudinal unstriped muscle fibres, which is situated between the membrana propria and the columnar epithelial cells. The glands that have this muscular coat are usually larger in size than the variety without it, and are especially well developed on the volar side of the hand and foot, axillæ, scrotum, labiæ, and scalp. They also occur by the side of the smaller glands. The ceruminose glands of the external ear passage are of the same structure as the larger variety, with the addition of yellowish-brown pigment granules in the epithelial cells. Sweat glands occur on all parts of the surface, but are more numerous on the palms and soles.

SEBACEOUS GLANDS.

The sebaceous glands are situated in the corium, and consist of gland substance and excretory ducts, which open usually at an acute angle into hair follicles, but occasionally upon the surface.

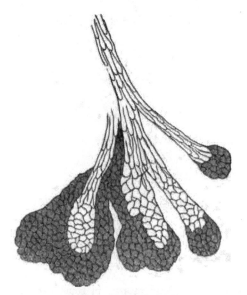

Fig. 5.—SEBACEOUS GLAND.

The gland substance is composed of lobules, filled with polyhedral cells, which open into the excretory ducts. A lobule is therefore a sac containing cells. The sac is a transparent and colourless nucleated membrane destitute of structure, and the cells are epithelial cells, the most external of which resemble those of the deeper layer of the rete Malpighii, some in the next layer contain drops of fat, whilst those in the centre of the sac are completely filled with the same substance. The cavity of the glands is occupied by fatty matter and the débris of the epithelial cells. The excretory duct consists of a transparent membrane and an epithelial investment, the cells of which correspond to those of the external root sheath, so that a sebaceous gland is really a protrusion of a hair follicle. The larger glands nearly surround the hair follicle, and are composed of several lobules. There are no sebaceous glands on the palm, sole, dorsum of the third phalanges, or glans penis, and the largest are found at the entrance of the nose, the lips, the labia externa, and the scrotum.

Hair Follicle.

This is a depression in the corium which has a blind inferior dilatation and a funnel-shaped excretory duct. The neck is

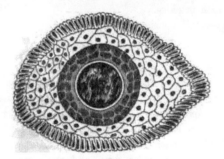

Fig. 6.—Transverse Section of Hair and Hair Follicle.

the contracted part below the duct where the sebaceous follicle opens. The follicle itself consists of two parts—

        1. The hair sac.
        2. The root sheath.

The hair sac consists of three layers—external, middle, and internal.

The external layer is composed of fibres of connective tissue which run parallel to the axis of the hair and join the fibres of the corium above, whilst below they encircle the dilated extremity of the follicle.

The middle layer is formed of transverse fibres of connective tissue, between which is a homogeneous, slightly granular material that contains numerous rod-shaped, transversely arranged nuclei. This layer is highly contractile. Between these two layers are situated two or more longitudinal blood-vessels, which by their free anastomoses form a network around the follicle. The papilla of the hair protrudes into the cavity of the follicle, and is constituted of connective-tissue fibres derived from this layer. The constricted portion of the papilla is the neck, and the thicker part the body, which has a conical extremity. The length is generally double the breadth.

The internal layer, thin and transparent, is a continuation of the basement membrane of the corium, and is called the vitreous membrane; the outer surface is smooth, whilst the inner is covered with prickles.

The root sheath consists of two layers—

      1. The external root sheath.
      2. The internal root sheath.

The external root sheath is a continuation of the rete Malpighii, which dips into the follicle, but terminates usually at a level with the apex of the papilla. The external layer of cells— viz. those that are in contact with the basement membrane—are columnar in shape, with nuclei at the inner extremity ; the cells of the next layer are polyhedral, and the most internal are flattened. The sheath is thinnest at the neck of the follicle, but becomes thicker towards the bulb, where in the hairs of embryos and children small, simple or compound, budlike prolongations of the cells are seen.

The internal root sheath consists of two layers—

      1. The outer or Henle's layer.
      2. The inner or Huxley's layer.

1. *The outer or Henle's layer* is a thin, transparent membrane, which commences at the neck of the follicle and extends as far as the external root sheath. The membrane is composed of oblong, non-nucleated, highly refractile scales in immediate contact with one another, which run parallel to the long axis of the hair.

2. *The inner or Huxley's layer* consists of flattened, fusiform, nucleated cells filled with small refractile granules. At the lower part of the follicle, and also towards the neck, the two layers are indistinguishable. The follicles of lanuginous hairs are so small that the relations between them and the sebaceous glands are reversed, and they appear merely appendages of the relatively large gland.

MUSCULAR TISSUE.

Striated muscular tissue is present in the skin of the face where it terminates in the corium.

A small involuntary muscle, called *arrector pili*, arises in the upper part of the corium, passes obliquely through it, and is inserted into the inner sheath of the hair follicle below the sebaceous gland; but some hair follicles have two muscles, which encircle the gland, and have a twofold action—to erect the hair and to compress the gland. There is, however, other involuntary muscular tissue in the corium, which runs either horizontally, as in the scrotum (dartos), or circularly, as in the nipple and in the areola around it.

HAIR.

A hair is divided into the shaft, which projects beyond the skin, and the root, which lies embedded in the hair follicle. The structure of a hair consists of cortical substance, with addition in some of the larger hairs of a central medulla composed of granular polyhedral cells.

A cuticle of homogeneous, transparent, non-nucleated scales, overlapping one another at their margins, encloses the cortical

part. The root, which terminates in the bulb, surrounds a
papilla projecting from the corium at the bottom of the follicle,
and is composed of nucleated cells resembling the deeper cells
of the rete Malpighii. The outer of these cells are flattened,
and the inner are columnar in form and rest upon the surface
of the papilla. In the root there is, besides the above-men-
tioned cuticle, another layer of flattened cells, which fits into
spaces between these and is continuous with Huxley's layer.
The cortical substance, which is colourless in grey hairs and
contains various-coloured pigment granules in other hairs, is
in the main portion composed of longitudinal fibres, which
towards the bulb appear as fusiform cells with rod-shaped
nuclei, and which at the transition into the bulb become
shorter and shorter until the polyhedral cells constituting the
bulb are reached.

Hairs grow by the multiplication of the cells of the bulb
lying next to the papilla. These new cells are gradually pushed
outwards by the formation of yet newer cells, and become more
fusiform as they leave the papilla. They also become more
elongated, owing, perhaps, to the pressure of the internal root-
sheath. Hairs are dissolved by strong solutions of potash.

NAILS.

The nails are horny, elastic, transparent, concavo-convex
laminæ embedded in the skin on the dorsal surface of the last
phalanges, and are composed of nucleated epidermic cells firmly
cemented together. They have an anterior, a posterior, and
two lateral borders, an upper convex and a lower concave surface, the latter of which is situated on what is called the bed of
the nail. This bed is formed by the rete Malpighii, the corium,
and the subcutaneous tissue below it.

The last contains no fat, and its fibres pass in separate
bundles from the periosteum of the phalanges backwards to the
posterior border or root of the nail. The anterior part of the
upper surface of the corium appears in ridges, consisting of

parallel fibres of connective tissue, between which lie numerous fusiform cells, and the posterior part is covered with small papillæ.

These ridges and papillæ contain loops of blood vessels which are connected with a coarse plexus in the corium. The rete Malpighii is much the same as in other parts, and is continuous with the root of the nail, but the stratum lucidum shows a distinct layer of granular cells.

BLOOD VESSELS.

The large trunks of both arteries and veins are situated in the deeper parts of the subcutaneous tissue, forming a coarse plexus, and branches of varying length pass from the former through the mass of the corium to supply the various structures already described. The length of the branches depends upon the position of the organs to be supplied, and all of them terminate in capillary networks, from which the veins take their origin. There are several special capillary networks.

1. For the papillary body, the papillæ of which contain vascular loops.
2. For the coiled tube of the sweat glands.
3. For the hair follicles and the arrectores pili.
4. For the sebaceous glands.
5. For the adipose tissue.

NERVES.

Sensory nerves, composed of both medullated and non-medullated fibres, arise from trunks that accompany the larger blood-vessels in the subcutaneous tissue. The medullated fibres pass through the corium, and either end in the special terminal organs or become non-medullated, and form a subepithelial plexus, from which certain fibrils enter the rete Malpighii, where they branch and form a delicate terminal network lying in the intercellular spaces. In a similar manner the nerves terminate in the outer root sheath of the hair follicle. The special terminal organs are—

    A. Pacinian corpuscles.
    B. End bulbs of Merkel.
    C. Tactile or Meissner's corpuscles.

A. *Pacinian Corpuscles.*—These corpuscles, which are oblong, elliptical, or pointed, consist of a number of capsules arranged concentrically around a central elongated clear mass. Each capsule is composed of a hyaline ground membrane, probably elastic, in which are embedded fine connective-tissue fibres, that lie transversely, and on its inner surface is lined by

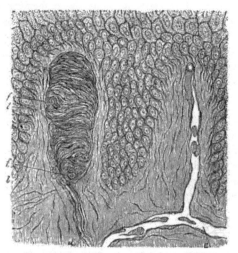

Fig. 7.—*a*, vascular ; *b*, nervous papilla ; *c*, blood vessel ; *d*, medullated nerve-fibre ; *e*, tactile corpuscle ; *f*, transversely divided medullated nerve-fibres. (After Biesiadecki.)

an endothelial membrane, formed of a single layer of flattened nucleated cells. The corpuscles are connected with medullated nerve fibres, which form the stalk, and are found most frequently in the subcutaneous tissue of the volar side of the hand and foot. The central clear mass is the axis cylinder of the nerve fibre, which usually divides into two or more branches, that terminate in pear-shaped or irregular bodies, called buds, and are composed of a dense network of minute fibrils. In some instances the corpuscle appears to have a second stalk, which is really an artery that ultimately divides into branches that give rise to a capillary plexus between the capsules.

B. *End Bulbs of Merkel.*—These are situated in the tissue of the papillæ or amongst the epithelium, and occur as single large and slightly flattened transparent nucleated cells enclosed in a capsule of connective tissue, and are in direct connection with the medullated nerve fibres.

c. *Tactile Corpuscles.*—These are oval bodies found in some of the papillæ, more particularly at the ends of the fingers. They, like the end bulbs, consist of a capsule, which contains a soft core composed of several small cells, and the termination of a medullary nerve-fibre.

LYMPHATICS.

The lymphatics of the skin are grouped into two systems, the superficial and the deep.

The superficial resemble lymphatic capillaries, as their walls are composed of a single layer of endothelial plates. They form a network in the superficial part of the corium in immediate vicinity to the rete Malpighii and parallel to the surface, and into it branches of varying length enter from the papillæ.

The deep lymphatics also form a network, which lies in the subcutaneous tissue, but the meshes are larger and possess the character of tubes to a greater degree than in the superficial plexus.

These two systems communicate by means of branches that are in immediate association with the blood vessels. The adipose tissue contains numerous lymphatics.

PHYSIOLOGY.

The skin serves some more or less important services in the economy, such as secretion, absorption, and tactile perception.

Secretion takes place in the form of perspiration by means of the sweat glands, which are continually carrying on their functions.

Perspiration is a clear, colourless, acid fluid, with a distinctive odour, that differs in various parts of the body. In a healthy man about thirty ounces is secreted in twenty-four hours, but this amount may be easily increased according to circumstances. For instance, more is secreted in summer than in winter, and more in consequence of exercise; certain foods and drugs also increase the flow, while at times mental emotion does the same. The perspiration that is perceptible to the sight is called sensible, and the portion that evaporates insensible. Perspiration consists chiefly of water, the average amount of solids being 1·81 per cent.

Constituents of Solids.

1. Sodium chloride and traces of other salts.
2. Fatty acids, such as formic, acetic.
3. Neutral fats and cholesterin.
4. Ammonia (urea), and possibly other nitrogenous bodies.

(*Foster*).

The amount of carbonic acid given off in twenty-four hours is from four to ten grammes, and the oxygen that is absorbed is rather less; however, the chief substance lost is water.

Animals that have been varnished soon lose heat, and die of some form of poisoning due to the absorption of some of the constituents of the perspiration. The skin has the power of absorbing, as is seen in the action on the system of certain drugs, like mercury and arsenic, after they have been well applied to the surface in a greasy form. The body also increases in weight by prolonged immersion in fluids.

For a description of the laws concerning the sense of touch the student is referred to the text books of Physiology.

c

J·9

CHAPTER II.

MORBID ANATOMY.

THE morbid processes which take place in the skin show themselves on its surface as certain discolorations, elevations, &c. These have received the name of the primary lesions. Enumerated, they are as follows :—

1. Macule.
2. Papule.
3. Tubercle.
4. Wheal.

5. Vesicle.
6. Bulla.
7. Pustule.

Hebra's definitions are—

1. *Macule.*—Any change in the normal colour of the skin, arising from disease, and not uniformly distributed over the whole surface of the body.

2. *Papule.*—Any morbid change in the skin which forms a solid projection above the surface, in size between a millet seed and a lentil, and containing within it no fluid.

3. *Tubercle.*—Any solid swelling of the skin, caused by disease, which contains no fluid, is as large as a lentil, bean, or hazel nut, and covered with epidermis.

4. *Wheal.*—A solid form of eruption slightly raised above the surface of the skin, of which the superficial area greatly exceeds the thickness.

5. *Vesicle.*—An elevation of the horny layer of the epidermis by transparent or milky fluid, corresponding in size to papules.

6. *Bulla.*—An elevation of the epidermis, in size between a

lentil and a goose's egg, containing transparent or yellow purulent fluid.

7. *Pustule.*—A small abscess, covered only with epidermis.

The process of ordinary inflammation of the skin is the sole
mode of production of such lesions as the wheal and bulla,
and is also the commonest cause of the other primary lesions.

In considering inflammation of the skin, it is necessary to
bear in mind a few facts as to its anatomy. There is the deep
plexus of vessels lying close beneath the level of the hair follicles, giving off branches, which in their turn break up to form
anastomotic networks round the follicle and sweat glands. From
it also communicating branches pass upwards to join the superficial plexus. The latter is situated beneath the papillæ, which
are freely supplied with branches from it. Owing to this
distribution of blood vessels in the skin, the papillary body, the
hair follicles, and the glands are the most vascular parts of the
integument, and as such are the first to give evidence of the inflammatory process.

Thus during the early stages of inflammation the dilatation
of the vessels and the increased blood flow give rise to hyperæmia of the part, which becomes visible through the epidermis.
The surface becomes red, and inflammatory macules are produced, which, according to their shape and distribution, constitute the eruptions known in this country as rashes.

Examples —Roseola, measles, erythema.

When the inflammatory process is confined to a minute
area, as round the orifice of a hair follicle, and when, in addition
to the hyperæmia, there is a further stage of inflammation present—viz. exudation into the substance of the papillæ—the inflammatory papule is formed.

Examples.—Lichen, papular stage of eczema.

If the above condition extends to an area larger than that
of a lentil, it is termed an inflammatory tubercle.

Example.—Erythema tuberculatum.

c 2

A similar state produces the wheal, but the inflammatory œdema of the papillary body is quite peculiar. The process is very acute, and the exudation readily re-absorbed; so that wheals are characterised by their transitory duration. In size they are, if discrete, about as large as the finger nail, or somewhat smaller, but may become much larger by confluence. They vary in colour according to circumstances, but for the most part are usually violet red. The presence, however, of the exuded fluid sometimes forces the blood from the vessels, and the wheal then becomes white. As this first takes place in the centre, it is not unusual to see white wheals with red margins. Wheals are generally irregular in outline. The process which gives rise to them is neurotic in origin, probably causes vasomotor spasm.

In the lesions hitherto considered the inflammatory exudation has not advanced beyond the true skin. In the vesicle, however, the serum transudes the boundary line between the rete mucosum and the papillæ, and making its way in the intercellular spaces, pushes the moist Malpighian cells asunder, and finally upheaves the horny layer of the epidermis. According to the extent of the area of epidermis raised by the exuded serum, a vesicle or bulla results.

Examples.—Vesicles, in herpes, vesicular stage of eczema ; bullæ, in pemphigus.

The transition from the vesicle to the pustule is merely the passage of the inflammatory process from a simple serous exudation to one accompanied by migration of leucocytes. Thus the fluid of vesicles is often seen to become milky, and afterwards straw-coloured, as the serum becomes richer in cells.

Example.—Impetiginous eczema.

Sometimes the inflammatory process subsides rapidly after having given rise to one or more of the primary lesions, such as papules and vesicles, and generally leaves behind it vestiges which may be traced for some time afterwards.

Whether the inflammation be transitory, whether it persists and becomes chronic, or is so by its nature from the beginning, certain secondary changes are set up in the tissues. As is well known, the epidermis derives its nourishment from the papillary body; consequently, congestion of the latter structure leads to a disturbance of nutrition of the epidermic cells; they do not pass through their chemical and physical changes, and are prematurely shed in larger or smaller masses as flakes or branlike scales. This is known as desquamation. It accompanies almost every inflammatory process, whether it be one which is of passing duration, as in measles, or whether it be chronic, as in psoriasis.

The next secondary change in the tissues resulting from inflammation is excessive deposit in the pigmentary layer of the epidermis, causing more or less brownish staining of the part, especially common in chronic inflammations. This change is known as pigmentation. There is another variety, not so permanent, which may accompany acute inflammatory conditions, and probably arises from the changes taking place in the exuded colouring matter of the blood, analogous to those seen in bruises.

An example of the first variety of pigmentation is well seen in chronic eczema, and of the second in some forms of old-standing urticaria.

A third change results from the increase of the cellular elements in the true skin, whether they be migrants from the blood or proliferated from the connective-tissue corpuscles already existing in the part. It seems that they ultimately lead, by a process of fibrillation, to an increase of fibrous tissue. Thus the corium and subcutaneous tissue become hypertrophied. The fold of skin thus affected is pinched up with difficulty from the subjacent tissues, and, on being compared with a fold of sound skin, the increase in substance is at once apparent.

This infiltration of the skin is well marked in chronic

eczema. It is almost always accompanied by pigmentation and desquamation.

There are certain changes, some of which affect the primary lesions themselves, which have received the name of secondary lesions; they are—

1. Scale.	4. Fissure.
2. Excoriation.	5. Scar.
3. Crust.	

The scale (*squama*) has already been discussed in connection with the process of desquamation.

The excoriation (*excoriatio*) is produced by the exposure of the moist rete by the removal of the horny layers of the epidermis. This happens when vesicles burst, or are ruptured by the violence of scratching or rubbing. It is not uncommon to see whole areas denuded of horny epidermis and exuding drops of serum from the exposed rete. This exudation soaks into linen in contact with the part and stiffens it, or it dries on the surface and gives rise to the secondary lesion known as the crust (*crusta*).

According to the character of the discharges crusts vary in appearance. Simple serous exudation gives rise to greyish leathery crusts; when there is pus the crusts are yellow, and may be brown, or even black, owing to a mixture of blood with the exudation.

The crusts that form on the head and face often have a peculiar honeylike appearance, due to the presence of sebaceous matter. Sometimes the affected surface, after having ceased to exude and commenced to desquamate, again becomes moist; the crusts and scales thus formed, alternately remaining adherent, are called *lamellated crusts*.

Crusts are best seen in eczema.

The fissure (*rhagas*) is nothing more than a crack in the skin. It may extend only to the epidermis, but more frequently it involves the corium. Fissures occur in skin which is rendered brittle by infiltration, and especially in parts which are subjected to much movement, such as the hands and flexures of joints.

The scar (*cicatrix*) replaces lost tissue. Scars indicate that the inflammatory process has been of the gangrenous variety— that is to say, it has been so severe that the cell production in the papillary body has caused strangulation of the vessels and consequent death of the part.

This variety of inflammation is characteristic of the disease variola, but it may occur spontaneously or as a result of continued irritation of the part in other affections—herpes, for example. Scars are white, smooth, devoid of hair follicles or glands. The appearance of a single scar furnishes no information as to its cause.

It has been shown how the process of ordinary inflammation of the skin may produce the so-called primary and secondary lesions, how its severity may cause loss of tissue, and how, when chronic, it leads to more or less permanent changes in the tissues.

Although the primary lesions, for the most part, correspond to certain types of inflammation, they cannot be regarded in any other light than that of evidencing so many stages in the inflammatory process, and as such they naturally pass from one into the other. Thus a disease which is generally characterised by the development of macules may present tubercles, or even bullæ, from the fact that an inflammation, which ordinarily stops at simple hyperæmia, has passed into one accompanied by exudation. Again, the eczematous inflammation commences in a papular eruption. Here it may cease; but more frequently the papules develope into vesicles, and these perhaps later on into pustules. A want of appreciation of the manner in which one type of inflammation passes imperceptibly into another has led to much confusion in dermatology.

There are certain specific inflammations of the skin, associated with diathetic conditions, such as syphilis, struma, and leprosy. These inflammations all commence in the substance of the true skin as small rounded cells, which are deposited in groups in the spaces of a fine reticulum, and are richly supplied with delicately-walled blood-vessels. From the great similarity of these deposits to ordinary granulation tissue, Virchow includes them all under the head of granulation growths. The deposits give rise to elevations on the surface, which, according to their size, are termed papules or tubercles; or they may be so superficial and diffuse as to appear like a simple macule. After a time the disturbance of the nutrition of the epidermis causes desquamation, and the tubercles are seen to be covered with scales. Unless interfered with by treatment, the tendency of these deposits of new growth is to increase until a point is reached at which their proper nutrition can no longer be maintained; they then break down and ulcerate; as they heal cicatrices are left, the result of the destruction of tissue which perishes with the new growth.

Some other modes of production of the primary lesions must now be briefly noticed.

A macule is defined as 'any change in the normal colour of the skin.' Besides the inflammatory macule we must include the discoloration caused by the escape of the colouring matter of the blood into the surrounding tissue, as seen in purpura. These purpuric macules are distinguished from the inflammatory by the fact that the colour does not disappear on pressure. Occasionally one variety passes into another. Small dotlike purpuric macules are called petechiæ. When once the colouring matter of the blood has entered the tissues, the part undergoes a characteristic series of changes in colour, as seen in bruises. There are white macules, due to absence of pigment in the skin, as in leucoderma, and brown, due to excessive deposit of pigment, as in liver-spot and freckle, or to parasitic growth, as in tinea versicolor.

Papules arise from many causes besides that already pointed out as resulting from inflammatory œdema of the papillæ. There are, for instance, the papules arising from minute lupus or sypbilitic deposit in the corium. They are also formed by a heaping up of the epidermis at the mouth of the hair follicle (*lichen pilaris*). There are conditions of the sebaceous glands which lead to the production of papules, as when they degenerate and form little white solid bodies protruding above the level of the skin, especially in the neighbourhood of the eyelids (*milium*).

A very important mode of forming papules is seen in lichen ruber, in which an over-growth of the cells of the external root-sheath of the hair is said to take place, and ultimately produces the flat-topped, umbilicated papule. There are also other less important varieties of papules.

All that applies to the papule may be said of the tubercle, the distinction between them being only the very artificial one of size. Tubercles either result from deposits of new growths (syphilis, lupus), or from a further development of smaller papules, as in the variety of erythema multiforme, known as erythema tuberculatum.

The wheal has already been discussed. Besides the vesicle of ordinary inflammation, which is best seen in eczema, it is said that there is another variety, produced in connection with the sweat duct in the condition known as sudamina. Vesicles which occur in situations where the epidermis is thick, as on the hands, acquire a peculiar sodden appearance at their margins, and are now known as the sago-grain vesicles.

Under the head of pustule must be included the catarrhal pustule, which often occurs as a further development of the vesicle, and also those suppurations round the hair follicles which result in small abscesses. Although the latter commence deep in the substance of the corium, the pus makes its way to the surface, and they ultimately appear as minute abscesses covered only with epidermis (acne).

The inflammatory bulla is seen in pemphigus. Other conditions give rise to the formation of bullæ, but chiefly as the result of accident (erysipelas, erythema multiforme). What may be termed false bullæ, as sometimes seen on the hands, are produced by the confluence of vesicles.

The foregoing remarks on the general pathology of the

skin will serve to show that for purposes of diagnosis the so-called primary lesions are, according to their definition, wholly useless.

First, because they may be caused by totally distinct conditions.

Secondly, because they may change as the process which gives rise to them becomes modified.

CHAPTER III.

CLASSIFICATION.

NEARLY every author who has written on skin diseases has suggested a new method of classification, based on some theory of supposed utility. The first system of any importance was founded by Willan, whose idea was to class the diseases under the heads of the more important external manifestations; thus he employed nine orders, each named after some particular symptom of an eruption, without paying any regard to the general character of the disease. For instance, varicella, herpes, and eczema are included in the order vesiculæ.

The next classification to be noticed is that of the French school, which is called the natural system, because the nature of the disease, and not the symptoms, forms its basis. This was introduced by Alibert, and modified later by Hardy, but has not been used to any great extent in this country.

The anatomical system was proposed by Erasmus Wilson, who grouped skin diseases into four principal classes—

1. Affections of the corium;
2. Of the sudoriparous glands;
3. Of the sebiparous glands;
4. Of the hair and follicles.

These classes are divided into several sub-classes.

The classification introduced by Hebra, and most frequently made use of in this country and in America, is founded on anatomico-pathological principles. He defines twelve classes—

1. Hyperæmiæ cutaneæ.
2. Anæmiæ cutaneæ.
3. Anomalies of the cutaneous glands.
4. Exudationes.
5. Hæmorrhagiæ cutaneæ.
6. Hypertrophiæ.
7. Atrophiæ.
8. Neoplasmata.
9. Pseudoplasmata.
10. Ulcerationes.
11. Parasites.
12. Neuroses.

Classification by cause would undoubtedly be the best, if sufficiently correct information could always be obtained; but in the present state of our knowledge of the subject such a plan is only partially possible. However, it will be seen that the last two classes in the following system are classified on this principle.

The system in this work is, in the first place, somewhat similar to Erasmus Wilson's in having two anatomical divisions; and, further, with certain slight modifications it resembles Hebra's in subdividing them into pathological classes.

Division I.—DISEASES OF THE SKIN PROPER.

Class I.—Exudationes.

Sub-class A.—Induced by Infection or Contagion.

1. Scarlatina	10. Equinia
2. Morbilli	11. Malignant pustule
3. Rötheln	12. Verruca necrogenica
4. Variola	13. Framboesia
5. Varicella	14. Erysipelas
6. Vaccinia	15. Septicæmic rashes
7. Typhus	16. Surgical rash
8. Enteric	17. Syphilis
9. Diphtheria	

Sub-class B.—*Of Internal or Local Origin.*

Erythematous .
1. Erythema . { Simplex, læve, fugax, intertrigo, multiforme, nodosum
2. Roseola
3. Urticaria
4. Pellagra

Papular .
1. Lichen . . { Simplex / Ruber and planus / Scrofulosorum
2. Prurigo . . { Of Hebra / Infantum, of Hutchinson / Recurrens   „

Vesicular and bullous
1. Herpes . . { Febrilis . / Gestationis / Iris
2. Pemphigus . { Vulgaris / Foliaceus

Eczematous and pustular
1. Eczema . . { Simplex / Rubra / Varieties (local)
2. Impetigo contagiosa (porrigo)

Squamous . . . . { 1. Pityriasis rubra / 2. Psoriasis / 3. Pityriasis

Phlegmonous and ulcerative { 1. Furunculus / 2. Anthrax / 3. Delhi boil / 4. Ulcers (varieties)

Class II.—VASCULAR.

Hyperæmiæ
Anæmiæ
Hæmorrhagiæ . . { Purpura simplex / „ rheumatica / „ hæmorrhagica / Scorbutus

Class III.—NEUROSES.

Zoster
Cheiro-pompholyx
Pruritus
Dystrophia cutis

Class IV.—HYPERTROPHIÆ.

Pigmentary . . . .
{ 1. Ephelis, lentigo
2. Melanoderma
3. Morbus Addisonii
4. Chloasma uterinum }

Epidermis and papillæ . . Iohthyosis, xeroderma

Connective tissue . .
{ 1. Morphæa
2. Scleroderma
3. Sclerema neonatorum
4. Elephantiasis arabum
5. Elephantiasis teleangiectodes
6. Dermatolysis }

Class V.—ATROPHIÆ. .

Pigmentary.. . . . { 1. Albinismus
2. Leucoderma }

Connective tissue . . Atrophia cutis

Class VI.—NEOPLASMATA.

Sub-class A.—*Benign.*

Papillomatous . . .
{ 1. Clavus
2. Tylosis
3. Verruca
4. Cornua }

Of connective tissue . .
{ 1. Keloid
2. Fibroma
3. Xanthoma }

Of granulation tissue . .
{ 1. Lupus . { Vulgaris
Erythematosus }
2. Rhinoscleroma }

Of blood vessels . . { 1. Nævus
2. Angioma }

Of lymphatics . . . Lymphangioma cutis

Sub-class B.—*Malignant.*

1. Lepra . { Maculosa
Tuberosa
Anæsthetica }

2. Carcinoma
3. Epithelioma
4. Ulcus rodens
5. Sarcoma.

Division II.—DISEASES OF THE APPENDAGES OF THE SKIN.

Subdivision A.—*Of the Sebaceous Glands.*

1. Seborrhœa
2. Acne punctata . { Nigra (comedo) Alba (milium)
3. Acne vulgaris
4. Acne sycosis
5. Acne rosacea
6. Molluscum contagiosum

Subdivision B.—*Of the Sweat Glands.*

1. Hyperidrosis
2. Anidrosis
3. Bromidrosis
4. Chromidrosis
5. Sudamina

Subdivision C.—*Of the Hair.*

1. Hirsuties
2. Lichen pilaris.
3. Nævus pilosus
4. Canities
5. Alopecia
6. Alopecia areata
7. Trichorexis nodosa

Subdivision D.—*Of Nails.*

1. Onychia
2. Onychogryphosis
3. Onychauxis
4. Onychatrophia
5. In general diseases

Class A.—PARASITIC AFFECTIONS.

Animal
- 1. Pediculosis
  - Corporis
  - Capitis
  - Pubis
- 2. Scabies
- 3. Eruptions from fleas, &c.

Vegetable
1. Tinea tonsurans
2. Kerion
3. Tinea sycosis
4. Tinea circinata
5. Eczema marginatum
6. Tinea versicolor
7. Tinea favosa

Class B.—ERUPTIONS PRODUCED BY DRUGS.

It will be noticed that although in the main we have followed Hebra, yet there are certain alterations in arrangement, due chiefly to the more recent researches in pathology. Much assistance has been gained from Dr. Bulkley's article on the subject in the ' Archives of Dermatology ' for April 1879, and many of his suggestions and names have been adopted.

DIVISION I.—DISEASES OF THE SKIN PROPER.

CHAPTER IV.

Class I.—EXUDATIONES.

Sub-class A.—*Induced by Infection or Contagion.*

SCARLATINA—MORBILLI—RÖTHELN.

ACUTE INFECTIOUS DISEASES.

THE acute infectious diseases agree in certain broad features. As a rule, each occurs but once in the history of an individual, one attack protecting the patient from a subsequent attack if he be exposed to the virus.

They all run an acute course, and are characterised, first, by an incubation period, or period of latency, from the time when the poison is received to the appearance of the first symptom of the disease; secondly, by the presence of symptoms of constitutional disturbance; and, thirdly, during some period of the disease by the existence of an eruption on the skin.

Each of these diseases reproduces itself in any susceptible person exposed to its poison, and never causes any of the other acute infectious diseases.

Varieties of the same disease, however, do not necessarily produce the same variety, for these modifications are due not to any special properties of the poison, but to some condition in the constitution of the person who receives it.

Although some epidemics are known to be more fatal than others, the difference between them is due not to any special

D

virulence of the disease, but depends altogether on the condition of the community into which the disease is introduced. Occasionally it is found that the members of a family are all attacked by a very severe form of scarlatina, contracted from the same person, but this occurrence must not be regarded as a proof of anything but a special susceptibility of the family to the influence of the disease.

When large numbers of persons are attacked, as in the case of schools, where family susceptibility can be eliminated, it is not found that the character of the disease is the same in all cases, although it may be derived from the same source.

Finally, it must be pointed out that, having regard to the infectiousness of the diseases in this category, their early recognition is a matter of great importance, in order that persons suffering from them may be isolated and the necessary steps be taken to disinfect the articles they have infected.

SCARLATINA—SCARLET FEVER.

Definition.—Scarlatina is an acute infectious disease characterised by the presence of a red rash on the body and extremities, and of redness and swelling of the fauces, accompanied by symptoms of constitutional disturbance.

Symptoms.—Between twenty-four hours and seven or eight days after the reception of the poison the patient is attacked by shivering, vomiting, headache, and sore throat. The soreness of the throat rapidly increases, and from twelve to thirty-six hours after the beginning of the constitutional symptoms a rash commences to appear on the the chest, neck, and wrists, whence it may extend over the whole body. The rash is generally at its height about the third or fourth day of the disease, then begins to fade, and disappears in about a week or ten days. This disappearance is followed by desquamation of the cuticle, which generally begins in the latter part of the second week, but may commence as the rash fades or not until the end of the sixth week. Desquamation occurs over the whole body, particularly

on the hands and feet, and is by no means limited to the site of
the eruption.

During the continuance of the rash the condition of the
fauces is characteristic; the whole mucous membrane is highly
injected, the papillæ of the soft palate are bright red and prominent, and the whole of the parts are more or less swollen.
Occasionally ulceration of the tonsils takes place, and the glands
of the neck are nearly always somewhat enlarged, and sometimes
suppurate. The tongue at an early stage of the fever is covered
with a white fur, through which the papillæ, which have become
red and swollen, show themselves, particularly at the edges, thus
giving the strawberry appearance well known as a symptom of
the disease. Later on, as the fever subsides and as the rash
fades, the tongue commences to desquamate, the fur is gradually
removed, leaving it of a bright red colour, with its papillæ
considerably enlarged, and gradually the bright redness fades
to a normal hue, the papillæ cease to be swollen, and it recovers
its usual appearance.

From the first symptoms of the disease the temperature is
higher than normal, and becomes still higher on each subsequent day until the third or fourth day, when a temperature of 103° to 104° is reached, the evening temperature being
usually higher than the morning by about a degree. At the
end of a week the temperature gradually falls, and by about
the tenth or fourteenth day has again become normal. The
pulse is considerably quickened, especially at night, when in
adults 120 pulsations often occur in the minute. During the
course of the disease the patient suffers from pain in the throat,
particularly in swallowing; he has severe headache, and frequently some delirium. At the height of the fever albumen is
often present in the urine, but disappears as the fever subsides;
at a later stage, however, especially about the end of the third
week, there is a tendency for it to reappear.

These are the symptoms of an average attack of scarlatina,
but it must be borne in mind that they are liable to considerable modification—that the rash may be absent, or may appear

D 2

only in a few dark patches or as a bright efflorescence over the whole body ; that the constitutional disturbance may be almost absent or may be of the severest character; that the condition of the throat varies with the severity of the attack from a simple injection to a condition ending in sloughing of tonsils, uvula, and cervical glands ; and that the delirium may be altogether absent, or present at night only in a mild form or in the most violent type.

It is now necessary to describe more particularly the varieties of rash which are present in the different forms of scarlatina.

In an attack of average severity the rash first appears on the chest and neck as minute red points, which are slightly raised, the skin intervening between them being of the normal colour. Later on they become brighter, and the redness which is at first limited to them extends over the intervening skin. If examined carefully, they can still be distinguished by the fact that they are redder than the surrounding skin. At this stage the skin is found to be rough on passing the hand over it. As the rash becomes more fully developed the identity of the red points is lost in the general hyperæmia ; but this stage is not always reached, and in the milder form of scarlatina this identity is not lost until the rash commences to fade, while in some rarer forms the eruption does not become confluent during its whole course. The distance between the spots varies in different parts of the body. On the chest, neck, and face they are so close as usually to become confluent, while on the wrists, backs of the hands, and dorsum of the feet they are farther apart, and more frequently remain separate than when situated on the chest and neck. In some cases the intense hyperæmia of the red spots causes minute vesicles to be formed at these points. These vesicles last but twenty-four or forty-eight hours, and when they dry up the skin desquamates freely.

In the most severe forms of scarlatina an entirely different eruption is present. Instead of bright red points appearing there is at once an escape of colouring matter from the capillaries into the superficial layers of the skin. This happens within twenty-four or thirty-six hours from the first symptom. A purple mottled appearance is thus produced, which but partially fades on pressure. There is slight general hyperæmia of the skin, but the rash is of a dusky red, which betokens an unfavourable termination. Accompanying this form in children there is the most intense restlessness and partial unconsciousness, while in adults complete consciousness sometimes remains, but there is constant vomiting of brown liquid from the stomach, a feeble, rapid, and compressible pulse, and a sense of extreme prostration. Between this and the milder forms of scarlatina there is every gradation, but it may be accepted generally that the tendency to hæmorrhage and the dusky colour of the rash is an indication of a severe form of the disease. In the most severe forms the tongue is spongy; later it becomes dry, glazed, and red, and finally cracks and bleeds.

The temperature in the hæmorrhagic form is not always specially high, often not reaching above 103°; but its chief characteristic is irregularity, a considerable fall often preceding the fatal termination, while in the death agony it rises, and even after death continues to rise.

Occasionally later in the disease, even as long as a month after the first symptom, the patient again suffers from sore throat, the fauces again become swollen and injected, albumen appears in the urine, and a rash once more is developed on the chest. This varies much in appearance, but usually begins as a number of minute red points, which are soon lost in a general hyperæmia. The rash lasts sometimes but twelve hours, sometimes two or three days, and is in all probability due to some septic condition.

During desquamation an occasional simple injection occurs on the chest, without the presence of any constitutional symptoms. It is not uncommon also, during convalescence, to find the legs covered with a mottled rash, which does not fade on pressure, due to the escape of blood colouring matter into the surrounding tissue. This lasts but a few days, and is also not attended by any constitutional symptoms.

Finally, it must be remembered that in all these rashes there is no tendency to œdema of the skin, except occasionally slight fulness or puffiness about the eyes, and that, with the exception of those specially mentioned, all fade on pressure.

Diagnosis.—Care is often required in the diagnosis of scarlatina, although in an attack of moderate severity its symptoms are sufficiently well marked to make its separation from other diseases a simple matter. It will not be necessary to refer to all the symptoms already described, but it will be sufficient to point out that at any period of the rash the disease may be recognised not only by the character of the eruption, but by the sore throat, the injected fauces, the strawberry character of the tongue, the pyrexia, and the constitutional symptoms.

In the most severe form, when no rash is present, the diagnosis of scarlatina is almost an impossibility. Vomiting and high temperature, succeeded by restlessness, delirium, and coma, are symptoms which are rather suggestive of poisoning than of a specific fever, but as a rule cases such as these do not occur singly, and other cases of less severity occurring immediately afterwards in members of the same family often throw light upon the first case.

In the hæmorrhagic forms the same difficulty also exists, but to a less degree, for in them the condition of the throat is often sufficient to aid the diagnosis.

From the hæmorrhagic form of variola—the disease for which it is likely to be mistaken during small-pox epidemics—it may be distinguished, first, by the implication of the throat; secondly, by the absence of pain in the back in scarlatina—an almost constant symptom of variola; and, thirdly, by the absence of the abortive papules and vesicles which can usually be found among the hæmorrhages in the latter.

From roseola it may be distinguished, first, by the smaller size of the red points in the rash of scarlatina, and by the fact that in scarlatina the skin intervening between these points soon becomes injected. The condition of the throat and tongue, as well as the presence of pyrexia, make the diagnosis between the erythemata and scarlatina a simple matter. Between a very mild form of scarlatina, in which the space intervening between the red points does not become injected, in which the temperature is but slightly raised and the throat but little affected, and roseola there is often much difficulty in diagnosis; but it must be noted that in scarlatina a larger extent of the soft palate and fauces are injected than in roseola, and that the enlargement of the papillæ of the tongue covers a larger surface than in the latter disease; moreover, the papules of roseola are more raised than the red points of scarlatina.

The accompanying table (p. 40) shows the distinctive symptoms of scarlatina, measles, and rötheln.

Prognosis.—The termination of a case of scarlatina can, as a rule, be correctly predicted after the rash has existed for twenty-four hours. Until this time a guarded opinion should always be given. When the rash is fully developed and of a bright red colour, when the throat affection is characterised more by injection than by swelling of tonsils and enlargement of cervical glands, when the pulse is not increased in adults to above 120 at night, recovery may be expected. When, however, the rash is badly developed and of a dark colour or hæmorrhagic, the pulse very rapid, and a tendency for the temperature to be very irregular, the mortality is very high.

In giving an opinion on the probable termination of a case of scarlatina, it should be borne in mind that the mortality is inversely proportionate to the age of the patient, children of two or three years of age dying in much larger proportion than those older. It may also be noted that ricketty children, as a rule, have much more severe attacks than others, and that they are more liable to suffer from severe throat affection and suppuration of glands.

Morbid Anatomy (abridged from Klein's 'Report to the Privy Council').—In scarlatina the morbid changes which take place in the skin are mainly those of hyperæmia and slight

	SCARLATINA.	MEASLES.	RÖTHELN.
Rash	Consists of minute red points close together on a bright red hyperæmic ground.	Consists of papules of larger size, arranged somewhat in crescentic manner on a white ground of normal skin.	Consists of slightly raised patches, varying in size, but usually about the size of a pea. The skin intervening between the spots is normal in colour or very slightly reddened, but later on the patches occasionally become confluent.
	First appears on chest, neck, and face.	First appears on forehead and face, and extends downwards.	First appears on chest.
	Appears after about 24 hours' illness.	Appears after about 72 hours' illness.	Appears first, or is preceded for a few hours by slight catarrh.
	Attended by marked injection of fauces, increase of temperature, strawberry tongue, slight suffusion of eyes.	Only slight sore throat and but little injection, high temperature, furred tongue, papillæ sometimes enlarged, but to a less extent than in scarlatina. Marked coryza.	Fauces injected, but less so than in scarlatina. Temperature slightly increased. Tongue furred.
	Followed by desquamation of skin in large flakes.	Occasionally by desquamation of skin in very small scales.	No desquamation, or only in the shape of small scales.
	Glands of throat enlarged.	Glands, as a rule, not enlarged.	Glands enlarged at different portions of body, and especially at back of the sterno-mastoid muscle.

exudation, with consequent nutritive changes in the epidermic layers.

1. The rete Malpighii, as a whole, is thickened, its cells separated by more or less fluid effusion, and leucocytes to a considerable extent are present. In some of the cells the nuclei are seen to be enlarged and constricted or double, indicating fission of the rete cells.

2. In later stages the rete is less thickened, but here and there local thickenings of the stratum lucidum, the cells of which are full of granules, and partial loosening of the stratum corneum are found, preceding the separation of large masses by desquamation. In the hair follicles the epithelium of the external root-sheath is often thickened, has its nuclei dividing, and contains some scattered leucocytes. The inner root-sheath is also thickened, more nucleated and granular. The epithelium of the sweat glands shows signs of germination, and is sometimes found loose in the tubes, having been detached by inflammatory exudation, which sometimes contains blood. Occasionally in S. maligna hæmorrhages occur into both the cuticle and the corium. The corium in early stages presents signs of inflammatory œdema, its papillæ are enlarged, the lymphatics and blood vessels well filled, and leucocytes present in abundance. In the blood vessels there is multiplication of the endothelial nuclei and of the muscle cells in the walls of the arterioles.

Treatment.—Inasmuch as scarlatina is an acute disease running a rapid course, the treatment consists in putting the patient under circumstances most favourable to his recovery. Thus a well-ventilated room of moderate temperature, the careful regulation of diet—which should consist simply of milk, beef tea, &c., during the pyrexial period—attention to the bowels, and, if necessary, in severe cases, when the strength is failing, the administration of stimulants, are as a rule sufficient. Delirium and sleeplessness, when present, are best treated with chloral hydrate and bromide of potassium. The frequent sponging of the body with water, vinegar, &c., is extremely useful. Severe pyrexia should be treated with cold baths. The patient should remain in bed for three weeks from the beginning of the disease, with a view to preventing kidney complication. Albumen, after two or three weeks' illness, should be constantly looked for, and the treatment regulated accordingly.

MORBILLI—MEASLES.

Definition.—Measles is an acute infectious disease characterised by the production of an eruption of red papules, accompanied by symptoms of coryza and general constitutional disturbance.

Symptoms.—From ten to fourteen days after the reception of the poison the patient becomes ill and feverish, shivers, sometimes vomits, and complains of headache. The skin becomes dry and hot, the tongue coated with white fur, through which a few large papillæ may show themselves; the eyes become suffused, the eyelids swollen, the fauces injected, and sneezing, pain in the frontal sinuses, and all the symptoms of a severe catarrh appear. The temperature rapidly increases, the pulse is quickened, and the rash appears on the fourth day, first on the forehead and face, and thence extends over the rest of the body and extremities, about one or perhaps two days being occupied in its complete development.

As the rash makes its appearance the face becomes more swollen, the coryza increases, and an exacerbation of the constitutional symptoms, together with some amount of bronchitis, nearly always appears. After the rash has existed for two or three days it gradually fades, and the constitutional symptoms subside.

The rash first presents itself as a number of small red spots irregularly scattered over the skin, which rapidly become raised, forming dark red-coloured papules from $\frac{1}{30}$ to $\frac{1}{4}$ of an inch in diameter.

On the face especially, and on all parts of the body where the papules are closely aggregated together, they coalesce and form patches of various sizes and of a crescentic shape; as the rash fades a temporary staining of the skin remains, which disappears after some days. The rash fades on pressure, but at once reappears on the removal of the finger, and its disappearance is often followed by desquamation of the skin in small scales.

Several varieties of the rash are described.

1. *Morbilli læves.*—In this variety healthy skin intervenes between the maculæ, which are but slightly raised.

2. *Morbilli papulosi.*—The papules are more raised and of a dark red colour; they are situated at the mouth of hair follicles, and closely resemble the papules of small-pox.

3. *Morbilli vesiculosi.*—The mouths of the hair follicles are filled with fluid, and small vesicles are thus produced.

4. *Morbilli confluentes.* — Occur when the maculæ are crowded so closely together that they coalesce and no healthy skin intervenes between them.

5. *Morbilli hæmorrhagici.*—This form of rash results from hæmorrhage into the maculæ, which of course do not then fade on pressure.

Diagnosis.—There are four diseases for which measles may at first sight be mistaken—scarlatina, rötheln, roseola, and variola.

The following table will show the difference between these diseases in the early stages; at a later stage the difference in the appearance of the rashes becomes more marked, the different constitutional symptoms more fully developed, and the diagnosis consequently easier :—

MORBILLI.	SCARLATINA.	RÖTHELN.
Rash appears on the fourth day.	Rash appears on the second day.	Rash appears on the first day.
Slight sore throat. Tongue furred, few papillæ enlarged.	Considerable sore throat and injection of fauces. Tongue furred, many papillæ enlarged.	Slight sore throat. Tongue furred; papillæ slightly enlarged, chiefly at edges.
Severe catarrhal symptoms.	No catarrh.	Slight catarrh.

ROSEOLA.	VARIOLA.
Rash appears on the first day.	Rash appears on the third day.
Slight sore throat. Tongue very slightly furred, only few papillæ enlarged at edges.	Slight sore throat. Tongue furred, papillæ not enlarged.
No catarrh.	Suffusion of eyes only.
	Severe lumbar pain.

Prognosis.—Usually favourable, but at times dangerous, owing to the long complication.

Morbid Anatomy.—On examining the measles eruption in its earliest stages, we find usually slight hyperæmia round the orifice of a sebaceous follicle, with slight swelling from effusion of plasma. Occasionally swelling alone is present, and more rarely the hyperæmia only. Round the minute hyperæmic papule thus formed (often with a hair in its centre) a roseolar patch, due to hyperæmia of the papillary body, soon appears. Slight exudation of plasma, with a few corpuscles, usually follows, and causes elevation of the papule itself. The pale brownish stain seen after the fading of the rash is due to changes in the escaped red corpuscles, and is deeper in proportion to the intensity of the previous congestion.

During the process of retrogression single or multiple reddish points, minute extravasations, may occur on the site of previous spots, or the hæmorrhages may appear more diffusely over the whole spot and have definite margins. These are due to local weakness of the blood vessels, allowing an easy escape of red corpuscles.

Occasionally the extravasations take place at the height of the rash, and remain after the papules have faded. Minute vesicles sometimes are seen in the centre of the spots, but they are met with chiefly in cases where profuse sweating is present, they are probably sudamina.

Treatment.—This consists in putting the patient on a proper regimen and paying careful attention to the bowels, &c. The lung complication may require the administration of an emetic and the application of warm poultices to the chest. Local treat-

ment of the rash is not required, but sponging the body with
aromatic vinegar and water is useful in allaying irritation.

Rötheln—German Measles.

Definition.—Rötheln is an acute infectious disease characterised by an eruption of red blotches on the skin, and attended
by slight sore throat, slight coryza, and but little constitutional
disturbance.

Symptoms.—After an incubation period usually of about
fourteen days, an eruption of oval or round spots, of a lighter
red colour than those of scarlatina or measles, appears on the
chest, afterwards extending over the rest of the body, which
vary in size from a pin's head to a threepenny piece. If the
spots be large they are generally irregular in their shape; if
small, they are more crowded together, and give an appearance
more resembling scarlatina. The spots are generally discrete,
but the rash is more often confluent on the face than on any
other part of the body. The rash lasts about two days, and
then fades, leaving a slight brown stain, which gradually dies
away; it is rarely followed by desquamation, and, if at all, only
in the form of minute scales. In rare cases the spots have been
known to become vesicular. The constitutional symptoms
which accompany the appearance of the rash are chiefly those of
catarrh, and occur at the same time as the rash, or precede it
by less than twelve hours, and not by some days, as in measles.
The fauces are somewhat injected, and the tonsils may be even
slightly swollen. The tongue is coated with white fur, through
which a few large papillæ can be seen, more often at the tip
than elsewhere. An important symptom which accompanies
the others is the tendency of the lymphatic glands to become
enlarged, which is more constantly the case in the neck, especially in those situated behind the sterno-mastoid muscle, but
the glands of other parts of the body are not always exempt.
Increase of temperature is rare in rötheln, or is limited to the
first few hours of the disease.

Diagnosis.—Rötheln may be confounded with three other affections—scarlatina, morbilli, and roseola. The chief characteristic points between rötheln and scarlet fever and measles are shown on p. 40 under the head of Scarlatina; from roseola it can be best distinguished by the absence of coryza in the latter disease, and by the glandular enlargement which occurs in the former. See also table, pp. 43, 44.

Prognosis is always favourable.

Morbid Anatomy.—The light red spots are due to capillary hyperæmia of the papillary layer, which very rarely goes on to slight exudation into the rete Malpighii, causing slight elevation of the spots. As they fade a very faint and transient pigmentation may remain, and minute epidermic flakes may be shed. The vesicles occasionally seen on the back are probably miliaria.

Treatment.—No special treatment is required.

CHAPTER V.

Class I.—EXUDATIONES—*continued.*

VARIOLA—VARICELLA—VACCINIA.

VARIOLA—SMALL-POX.

Definition.—An acute infectious disease characterised by the existence of a rash, which passes through the successive stages of papules, vesicles, and pustules, accompanied by symptoms of considerable constitutional disturbance.

Symptoms.—On the fourteenth day after the reception of the poison, headache, nausea, feverishness, severe lumbar pain, and general *malaise* are experienced. After forty-eight hours—that is, on the third day of the disease—an eruption of red papules appears on the face, especially its upper part, and on the wrists, then extends over the chest and back and the limbs generally; about two days are occupied in the gradual appearance of the rash.

The actual site of the spots is round a hair follicle or the orifice of sebaceous or sweat glands. The papules are frequently arranged in threes and fives in a crescent shape, two crescents often coming together to form a circle. A few hours after the first appearance of a red spot it gradually becomes elevated, increases in size, assumes a dark red colour, and is hard or 'shotty' to the touch; on the third day of the eruption the summit of the elevation becomes vesicular, and gradually, as the whole elevation takes this character, the summit becomes depressed, till on the fourth or fifth day of the eruption an umbilicated vesicle is formed, containing clear fluid. All the vesicles are not, however, umbilicated, this condition apparently depending on their being formed round the opening of a hair follicle. The contents of the vesicles gradually become more turbid, and by about the sixth day of the eruption become pustular. The base of the pustule then becomes hard, and the whole of the skin, especially about the face, becomes œdematous. About the eighth or ninth day of the eruption the pustules, which in the meantime have largely lost their umbilication, burst, and crusts or scales form on the surface. After a variable time, of from a few days to five or six weeks, the crusts are shed, and a depressed purple stain alone remains to indicate the position of the former pustule; from this a succession of fine scales are frequently shed. The colour may persist for some weeks, but gradually fades, and the depression contracts, leaving a cicatrix, the well-known 'pitting' of small-pox.

If the pustules have been numerous the skin of the face rarely recovers its normal pink, transparent appearance, but remains permanently of a uniform pasty white colour. During convalescence small abscesses frequently form in the skin, chiefly on the thighs and legs.

During the whole course of the disease the constitutional symptoms are severe. The temperature is increased to about 104°, 105° Fahrenheit, the tongue is covered with thick creamy fur, severe pains in the head and limbs, and especially in the back, are constantly present, while delirium, sometimes of the most violent character, and intense itching of the skin during the whole course of the eruption, prevent sleep, which is much required. As the crusts are formed the fever decreases until the temperature becomes normal. The severity of the constitutional symptoms depends altogether on the amount of rash. It has been stated that considerable variation exists in the different forms of small-pox; these will now be described.

1. *Variola discreta.*—The pustules remain separate from each other during the whole course of the disease.

2. *Variola semi-confluens.*—A few pustules run together on the face.

3. *Variola confluens.*—The pustules run together all over the body.

4. *Variola corymbosa.*—The pustules are arranged in groups, the skin surrounding which is free from eruption. This is a rare and fatal form of the disease.

5. *Variola hæmorrhagica.*—In this, the most severe form of variola, there is a bruised appearance.

The character of the bruises is such that it would be impossible to distinguish them from those produced by blows. But at the same time there is hæmorrhage beneath the conjunctivæ, and bleeding from nearly all the mucous membranes of the body. In this form, although there is great prostration, the mind is clear. The tongue is thickly covered with white fur, and the lumbar pain is severe. Often the attack is fatal before the appearance of the rash, but if not the papules appear rather as small hæmorrhages into the skin with ill-defined margins.

If the vesicular stage be reached the vesicles have irregular margins, which are obscured by the hæmorrhage, and the fluid which they contain becomes black from the presence of colouring matter from the blood.

The characteristic papules of small-pox may be preceded by a petechial rash. This consists of a quantity of minute petechiæ, closely aggregated together, which do not fade on pressure; their most frequent site is the lower part of the abdomen and the inner side of the thighs, the axillæ, the upper part of the arms, and the skin over the clavicle. The whole of the surface affected presents a dark and mottled appearance.

This rash must not be confounded with the true variola hæmorrhagica; often, however, the two are combined, and in these cases dark purple or rather blue bruises appear among the petechiæ; if there be no bruises—that is, if the rash be purely petechial and not hæmorrhagic—the petechiæ in a few days gradually fade, and are replaced by the true papules of variola, which appear while the petechiæ are still present. Sometimes the papules are preceded by a hyperæmia of the skin, which may be diffuse or in separate spots, and the disease then presents an

E

appearance closely resembling scarlatina, which is sometimes called variola roseola. The site of this rash is not limited, as in the petechial variety, but may occur over the chest and arms. It is not uncommon to see the roseolous and petechial rashes combined in the same individual, but they more often appear separately ; both usually commence on the second day of the disease.

Finally, it must be remembered that small-pox often occurs in persons who have been previously vaccinated, and that under these circumstances the course of the disease is greatly modified. The successive stages of development of the rash are more rapidly completed, the rash is far less abundant, and the constitutional symptoms are less marked.

Diagnosis.—The diagnosis of variola in the early stage is not so easy as in the later.

The roseolous rash may be mistaken during the first forty-eight hours both for scarlatina and roseola. Other symptoms, arranged in the following table, assist even at this early period in distinguishing between these diseases.

Symptoms during First Forty-eight Hours.

VARIOLA.	SCARLATINA.	ROSEOLA.
Very slight sore throat.	Severe sore throat.	Very slight sore throat ; redness limited to edge of soft palate.
Tongue furred.	Tongue furred.	Tongue slightly furred.
Papillæ not enlarged.	Papillæ enlarged.	Papillæ enlarged only at edges.
Rash of short duration.	Rash may last some days.	Rash of short duration.
Severe pains in back.	No marked pains in back.	No marked pains in back.
Pyrexia and constitutional symptoms.	Pyrexia and constitutional symptoms.	Pyrexia and constitutional symptoms subside with appearance of rash.

On the third day, when the papular rash is appearing, it

may be mistaken for measles, but it must be remembered that the rash appears on the third day in small-pox, and on the fourth day in measles, and that in the latter the chief constitutional symptom is coryza, whereas in the former there is only slight suffusion of the eyes and the usually well-marked lumbar pain. In a few hours the characteristic feeling of shotty papules, observable in passing the hand over the rash, makes the diagnosis of small-pox more simple.

A not uncommon mistake is to confuse acne, when accompanied by a pyrexial attack, with small-pox. Simple as the diagnosis apparently is, the two diseases are occasionally confounded, and it is well, therefore, to point out that the date of the appearance of the acne and the absence of the special constitutional symptoms of small-pox must be borne in mind. The same rule will enable small-pox to be distinguished from a secondary papulo-vesicular syphilide, for which it has sometimes been mistaken.

At a later stage the vesicles of small-pox present an appearance which prevents the disease being mistaken for any but varicella. Here, however, it should be remembered that the varicella rash appears on the second day, and in a few hours becomes vesicular, while in variola the date both of the appearance and vesiculation of the rash is later. The small, round, watery appearance of the varicella vesicle, its almost invariable freedom from umbilication, its tendency to appear in successive crops, scattered not in twos and threes but irregularly, renders the diagnosis anything but difficult.

Prognosis.—This will depend largely on the character of the rash.

The hæmorrhagic form is always fatal. The presence of the roseolar or petechial rash is not prognostic of anything special. The amount of rash is a most important sign, the danger depending directly on the amount. The discrete variety is not usually fatal, the mortality being about two or three per cent. among the unvaccinated. In semi confluent small-pox the mortality is about twice that of the discrete.

In variola confluens among the unvaccinated about half die. In the pustular hæmorrhagic form, where there is darkening of the vesicles, or if the vesicles be badly developed, the mortality is even higher. Age is also an important element, the mortality being much greater among the very young and old than among persons of middle age.

Morbid Anatomy.—In the first stage the variola spots consist merely of localised hyperæmic patches, in which there is slight serous infiltration of the papillæ.

In the papular stage the greater part of the little hard swelling is due to an increase in the thickness of the cells of the stratum lucidum, which undergo swelling and segmentation.

In the vesicular stage it is seen, on examining sections under the microscope, that the pock presents a chambered structure, most marked in its upper portion. It probably arises, according to Rindfleisch, through the serous infiltration of the epidermis not raising the horny layer *en masse,* as in a simple vesicle, but forcing its way gradually in between the lamellæ. It thus pushes asunder and displaces them from a horizontal to an oblique or vertical position. The fine filaments seen in the lower part of the vesicle may possibly be the remains of the cementing substance of the epidermis. The umbilicus seen in the centre of many of the vesicles is usually obviously due to the presence of hair follicles or the ducts of sweat or sebaceous glands, the tissues of which, being more resistant, act as bridles holding down the centre of the pock. It is not met with in every vesicle, and usually disappears at the stage of suppuration.

In the suppurative stage the papillary layer and the subjacent part of the corium are richly infiltrated with leucocytes, which escape freely into the vesicle. When mature, the umbilicus and most of the septa in the centre have melted away, and the pock consists of a somewhat irregular cavity filled with pus, mingled with epithelial débris.

In the process of drying up, or scabbing, the hyperæmia and exudation diminish; the rete cells at the margins and base of the pustule begin to cornify, and gradually form a fresh horny layer, which covers the papillæ, denuded, but not destroyed, and forms a closed capsule round the little pus mass; this dries up and is cast off. In some cases, however, the exudation of leucocytes, being excessive, separates the fibres of the papillæ widely, and pressing on the vessels, cuts off their blood supply and produces necrosis. Hence the base of the pock is formed by a pale slough, which has to be cast off by the suppuration around it. The tissue thus destroyed is replaced by granulations, which heal by second intention and leave a permanent scar.

In variola hæmorrhagica the hæmorrhages affect all the layers of the skin, and often the subcutaneous tissue also; they are probably due to transudation of corpuscles rather than to rupture of vessels, as no morbid condition has been detected in the latter. The hæmorrhages proceed not from the capillary plexuses round the hair follicles and glands, but from the loops in the papillæ at their apices or in their substance, as well as in the subjacent cutis.

During the stage of desiccation, since the centre of the pustule begins to dry up before the margin, an umbilicus is again formed even in pocks where it was at first absent.

Treatment.—This consists in putting the patient upon a suitable diet, placing him in a well-ventilated room, attending to his bowels, seeing that he gets sufficient sleep, and, when necessary, administering stimulants. With a view to prevent pitting, many applications and methods have been used; solution of nitrate of silver carbolic acid solutions, painting with collodion, powdering with fuller's earth, pricking and emptying the vesicles, have all in turn been resorted to, without any favourable result.

The application of oil to the surface is, however, useful in allaying the intense itching which accompanies the rash, and care should be taken to prevent the patient wounding the vesicles by scratching.

When the scabs form, if they be large they will often retain pus; they should then be softened with a poultice and removed. Abscesses should be opened early.

VARICELLA—CHICKEN POX.

Definition.—Varicella is an acute infectious disease, characterised by the production on the body of small round vesicles, appearing in successive crops. These dry up and form scabs, which fall off, sometimes leaving cicatrices.

Symptoms.—About a fortnight after the reception of the poison a crop of small roseolar papules, varying in number from a dozen or so to several hundred, appear first on the upper part of the body—usually the face—and are scattered irregularly over the surface, but not in twos and threes, as in variola. Within a few hours the papules become vesicular, and the rash is then usually described as having at this period the appearance of having been produced by a number of small drops of scalding water thrown on the skin.

The vesicles are of small size, usually less than one-fifth of an inch in diameter, filled with clear fluid, giving them a bright, glistening appearance, and seldom have a central depression. After twenty-four hours the vesicles become slightly turbid, and at the end of two or three days are covered with scabs. Later these separate, occasionally leaving pitting of the skin. On the first day of the rash about a dozen or fifteen vesicles appear; on the second day there may be as many as 100 to 150; and successive outbreaks occur during the first four or five nights. The rash is never confluent, but occasionally two vesicles may coalesce.

The eruption is generally attended with considerable itching and some constitutional disturbance, which is never severe. The temperature rarely rises above 100° Fahrenheit. The constitutional symptoms seldom precede the rash by more than a few hours, and usually occur simultaneously with it.

Diagnosis.—There is only one disease for which varicella can ever be mistaken, and that is variola. The differences between the eruptions will be found on p. 51. It may be well to mention that a vesicular syphilide has been occasionally mistaken for varicella, but to distinguish the two diseases it will only be necessary to point out that the syphilitic eruption rarely appears without other syphilides being present. The history and course of the two affections will serve to confirm the diagnosis.

Prognosis.—Favourable.

Morbid Anatomy.—On a small roseolar papule, due to superficial hyperæmia of the cutis, a small loculated vesicle soon forms. On examining this microscopically the cells of the upper layer of the rete are found filled with numerous refracting globules, scattered through the protoplasm and undergoing vesicular transformation. These cells, opening into one another, give rise to an irregularly loculated cavity, situated between the horny and the deeper layers of the rete, containing serous fluid, in which leucocytes and multinucleate epidermic cells float. As the cells undergo fatty degeneration, the clear serous fluid soon becomes turbid, and is absorbed, leaving a small brownish crust. On the separation of the scab there is left merely a slight depressed stain, which fades in time, leaving no trace unless suppuration and superficial ulceration of the papillary layer have taken place.

Treatment.—No specific treatment is required; the constitutional symptoms may be treated on general principles. The irritation of the skin is relieved by the application of oil. If suppuration occurs beneath the scab, the pus should be set free by poulticing.

VACCINIA—VACCINATION.

Definition.—An acute infectious vesicular disease of the cow, communicable to man, and which has the effect of protecting the latter from attacks of small-pox.

Symptoms.—With the disease in the cow we have here no concern, and therefore shall only describe the rash produced in the human subject by the inoculation of the cow pox in a person who has not previously been vaccinated. If a puncture be made in the skin of such a person with a lancet, and the vaccine matter be inserted with care, after two days, during which nothing appreciable occurs, a papular elevation is produced. On the fifth or sixth day this becomes a pearl-coloured vesicle of a round or oval form, depressed in the centre and with its edges raised. On the eighth day the vesicle is more distended, but the depression in the centre still remains. On the seventh or eighth day a red ring is formed round the vesicle, which may be two or three inches in diameter. The redness fades on pressure, but the area is harder and more tender than the surrounding skin. About the tenth day the redness begins to disappear, and the lymph in the vesicle is seen to become thick and purulent, while the umbilication is less marked. At the end of a fortnight a scab forms, which remains adherent till about the end of the third week, when it falls off, leaving in its place a somewhat circular depression, which is foveated. These pits correspond with the cells of the vesicles. The cicatrix contracts somewhat, but otherwise, as a rule, remains for life.

Two or three days after the operation considerable itching of the part is experienced, and about the seventh or eighth day there is usually, especially in young children, some amount of constitutional disturbance, such as shivering, loss of appetite, and general *malaise*. At this period the temperature is sometimes slightly increased; sometimes also the axillary glands become enlarged.

Although this is the course of by far the majority of the cases of vaccination, some are from time to time found which do not run through quite the same symptoms as described above. Thus occasionally a rose rash (*Roseola vaccinia*) makes its appearance between the third and eighteenth day after inoculation, commencing most often in the neighbourhood of the irritation and extending over other parts of the body. This rash consists of very slightly raised spots of a red colour, varying in size from a quarter of an inch to three or four inches in diameter. It lasts but a day or two, and is not followed by desquamation or deposit of pigment.

In *Variola vaccinia herpetica* a crop of vesicles appears on the third day after the operation, and is preceded by an attack of shivering. They soon burst; the fluid which escapes irritates the adjoining skin, and an eczematous condition of the part is produced, the skin becoming hard and œdematous. Intense itching accompanies this outbreak, and the axillary glands often become enlarged.

In *Variola vaccinia bullosa* a bulla of variable size, with a red edge, takes the place of the ordinary vesicle. It contains a clear liquid, which soon escapes, leaving a crust, which is shed without producing a scar, unless ulceration takes place, when the cicatrix is of considerable size.

In *Variola vaccinia furunculosa* red tubercles are formed, which subsequently suppurate.

Occasionally *Erysipelas* appears about the seventh to the tenth day round the vesicle, and spreads over the arm. It does not differ from ordinary erysipelas, and is accompanied by œdema, pain, and considerable constitutional disturbance. In some cases the pustules, instead of drying up and forming scabs, burst, and ulceration takes place. The ulcers are attended by itching, pain, and constitutional disturbance. This condition rarely results from lymph which has passed through the human subject, but occurs more frequently after inoculation direct from the cow.

But one other variety has to be described—that in which perfect vesicles are never developed, but scabbing occurs after a little fluid has been formed. It may be well also to mention that re-vaccination produces vesicles the typical characters of which are less marked, appearing earlier and running a more rapid course than in primary vaccination.

Vaccino-Syphilis will be noticed under ' Syphilis,' p. 96.

Prognosis.—A favourable result always follows vaccination, except in the rare cases when erysipelas occurs among young children.

Morbid Anatomy.—The structure of the vaccinal exanthem, in its successive stages of papule, vesicle, and pustule, is much the same as in variola.

The umbilicus of the vesicle is formed at the point of puncture, and is said to be due to the inflammation excited by the scratch causing adhesion of the corium and epidermis, so that the subsequent serous effusion separates the cuticle around the band thus formed. The vesicle is loculated, and, like that of variola, its umbilicus may disappear when suppuration sets in. Scabbing takes place in the centre and extends to the margin of the pock.

Treatment.—Vaccination requires but little treatment. The vesicles should be carefully protected from injury, and oil should be applied to allay the itching. On the eighth day, if the vesicles be much distended, a few punctures into them is useful to relieve tension. If there should be any tendency to retention of pus or ulceration beneath the scabs, they should be removed by a poultice, and the wound treated according to the rules for treating ulcers. If the erythema be great, or if erysipelas occur, the arm should be kept in a sling and lotio plumbi should be applied to the part.

Finally, it should be borne in mind that lymph should never be taken, for the purpose of vaccination, from any but a perfect vesicle, with a proper areola, in the person of a healthy child vaccinated for the first time.

CHAPTER VI.

*Class I.—*Exudationes*—continued.*

TYPHUS—ENTERIC—DIPHTHERIA.

Typhus Fever.

Definition.—Typhus is an acute infectious disease characterised by the production of a mottled rash, which becomes petechial, and which is accompanied by considerable constitutional disturbance.

Symptoms.—Thirteen or fourteen days after the reception of typhus poison there is a sense of chilliness and headache, accompanied occasionally by vomiting, and general pyrexial symptoms. On the third day, more often on the fourth or fifth, the mulberry rash of typhus makes its appearance. The rash can be described as consisting of two parts. The one which is simply an indistinct dark mottling appears as if it were a little distance beneath the surface of the skin, and is described as the 'subcuticular' mottling. The other consists of a quantity of small purple maculæ scattered over the surface of the skin, and appear to be altogether on the surface. When they first appear they are very slightly raised, but in a few hours become perfectly flat. The subcuticular mottling may exist by itself, but the maculæ are usually present as well. The rash is fully developed in less than forty-eight hours from its commencement, and no rash is ever produced after this period. For the first few days the spots fade on pressure, but later on a yellow stain is left, and still later pressure produces no effect on the spot, which has then become petechial; the petechiæ remain, appearing like minute hæmorrhages, and often last as long as three weeks,

but the mottling disappears earlier. The rash appears first on
the wrists, upper part and sides of abdomen, and about the
edges of the axillæ; later it gradually extends over the whole
abdomen and chest. The constitutional symptoms steadily
increase, especially the delirium, which is often of a violent
character. The tongue, which is first coated with white fur,
becomes dry, brown, and sometimes black, and great difficulty is
experienced in protruding it, on account of sordes collecting
about the mouth. Later the tongue begins to moisten at the
edges, and the appetite rapidly returns, even before the tongue
has cleaned. During the whole course of disease the temperature is raised constantly to 104° or 105° Fahr. The maxi-
mum temperature is usually reached on the fourth day, when
a slight fall takes place; a further fall occurs about the seventh
day, and although at the beginning of the second week it is
slightly lower than during the first, it rises until the crisis
occurs. This takes place generally between the twelfth and
seventeenth days. The temperature then falls rapidly, and
becomes normal within three or four days of the crisis, unless
some complication be present.

Occasionally erysipelas and glandular swellings, especially
of the parotid, occur during the course of the fever.

Diagnosis.—Typhus is frequently mistaken for brain disease, pneumonia, measles, and enteric fever. In the first two it
is only necessary to point out that no rash exists; from measles,
however, the diagnosis is not always an easy matter. In both
the rashes appear on the same day, but differ in certain essential
particulars (see table).

The diagnosis of typhus from enteric fever is a perfectly
easy matter, and a mistake should never be made between these
two diseases (see table).

Prognosis.—The chances of recovery depend altogether upon
age. The young nearly always recover, while among those of
middle or advanced life the mortality is very high. Fat, heavy
persons are more likely to die than those who are more spare.
A large amount of rash, which soon becomes petechial, especially

TYPHUS.	MEASLES.	TYPHUS.	ENTERIC.
Rash not very often present on face.	Rash commonly present on face.	Commences suddenly. Rash on fourth or fifth day.	Commences insidiously. Rash at end of first week.
Maculæ smaller than measles, separate from each other, and not raised.	Maculæ often coalesce and are raised.	Dark, mottled, non-elevated rash.	Group of lenticular roseolous papules.
Sub-cuticular mottling present.	Sub-cuticular mottling not present.	Rash fully developed in forty-eight hours.	Rash appears in successive crops, each spot lasting two or three days.
Suffusion of eyes, but no coryza.	Coryza.	Rash becomes petechial.	No petechiæ.
		Diarrhœa less common than in enteric.	Diarrhœa common.
		Flat abdomen.	Full, tender abdomen.
		Heavy, dull expression of face.	Flushed cheeks, glistening eyes.

if it be of a dark colour, an absence of fall of temperature at some period during the first week, a sudden rise of temperature during the third week, a very rapid pulse, much delirium, coma, convulsions, and suppression of urine, are all unfavourable signs.

Morbid Anatomy.—The rash of typhus is due to superficial hyperæmia of the cutis, but, as exudation is absent, the spots remain on a level with the rest of the skin. At a later stage the darkening of the spots is produced by the escape of red blood corpuscles from the vessels, and actual petechiæ sometimes form. These subsequently undergo the same changes as purpuric spots.

Treatment.—This should be regulated on general principles.

ENTERIC OR TYPHOID FEVER.

Definition.—Enteric or typhoid fever is an acute infectious disease characterised by swelling and subsequent ulceration of the Peyer's and solitary glands of the ilium, usually accompanied by successive crops of rose-coloured papules, chiefly on the abdomen, together with abdominal symptoms and considerable constitutional disturbance.

Symptoms.—From ten to sixteen days after the reception of the poison, headache, chilliness, and occasionally shivering, followed by a little delirium, are experienced. With these symptoms there is increased temperature, a furred tongue, and sometimes diarrhœa, or more often irregularity of the bowels, a few days of constipation being followed by purging. On the seventh, or from that to the twelfth day, in cases where a rash is present, a crop of round rose-coloured papules, from half a line to two lines in diameter, make their appearance on the abdomen, chest, and back. These are slightly elevated, and disappear on pressure, but reappear the moment the finger is removed. Their number varies from two or three to a hundred or so, but usually not more than about half a dozen are present at a time. Each crop lasts from three to six days, and is usually followed by subsequent crops. When the papules fade, no discoloration of the skin remains, and the rash is never permanent. The duration of the rash is from one to three weeks, but occasionally recurs at a later date if there is a relapse.

During the course of the disease the abdomen becomes prominent, and often tympanitic and tender on pressure, especially in the right iliac fossa, where it often produces gurgling.

The constitutional symptoms increase in severity after the first week, and sometimes the delirium is violent in character. The tongue becomes drier as the fever progresses, and towards the latter part of the second week is dry, very red, and glazed. Diarrhœa becomes a more common symptom in the second week, and is sometimes very severe. The stools are liquid and of a yellow-ochre colour. If allowed to stand, the more solid portion settles to the bottom, and is then found to consist of shreds of undigested food mixed with sloughs and débris from the ulcers in the intestine. Often they contain a little blood. In some cases severe hæmorrhage occurs from the ulcers, and the stool then consists almost wholly of blood.

At a later stage of the fever the ulceration of the intestinal glands occasionally extends through the peritoneum, and perforation of the intestine, with its accompaniments of extravasation into the peritoneal cavity and consequent peritonitis, results. The temperature in enteric fever is always increased during the first week; it rises higher and higher until a temperature of 104° Fahr. is frequently reached. The morning temperature is lower than the evening, and during the second and third week this is maintained. Later, however, usually in the third week, as the recovery begins, the difference between the morning and evening temperature is much more marked. Occasionally a sudden fall of temperature takes place, due usually to hæmorrhage from the bowel; but if any rise be observed, it is due to some complication, often of the lung. The pulse is always increased in enteric fever, often 120 at night, but less frequent in the morning.

In the mild cases the patient begins to recover at the latter part of the second week, and in more severe cases at a later date. Convalescence is always slow. Among the complications are hæmorrhage from the intestine, perforation of intestine, peritonitis, and pneumonia.

Occasionally two or three days before the lenticular spots make their appearance they are preceded by a scarlet rash, which spreads over the whole body. It is a mere temporary hyperæmia, and fades on pressure.

In rare cases petechiæ and purpuric spots occur during the course of the fever; they are in no way associated with the lenticular spots.

Taches bleuâtres are sometimes observed. They consist of blue patches, from two or three to eight lines in diameter, of irregular shape, usually separate, but sometimes coalescing. They are not raised, and give an appearance somewhat resembling the typhus spots, but they do not pass through the same changes as the latter. They are usually situated on the abdomen, thighs, and back.

Sudamina frequently occur, and are followed by desquamation.

Diagnosis.—The diagnosis of enteric fever is usually not a difficult matter. The high temperature, the prominent abdomen, the dry red tongue, the diarrhœa, and, when present, the lenticular spots, conclusively point out the disease. It can be recognised by the flushed cheeks, glistening eyes, and parched lips, which contrast strongly with the heavy, dull, leaden appearance of typhus, and by other symptoms, which are given in a tabular form on p. 61.

Prognosis.—Young children rarely die of enteric fever, but as age progresses mortality increases. A very high temperature which is not attended with morning remissions, much diarrhœa, hæmorrhage, tympanitis, delirium of a violent character, much muscular tremor, are unfavourable indications. The amount of rash is not prognostic of a favourable or unfavourable termination.

Morbid Anatomy.—The enteric papule begins as a small, circumscribed pink spot, due to hyperæmia of the papillary layer. In a day or two it becomes slightly raised, owing to the exudation of plasma into the papillæ and rete, and in some cases a minute vesicle, due to further collection of serum, forms at its apex. As the spot fades the plasma is absorbed, and the faint brown stain left by it soon disappears. The anatomy of the *taches bleuâtres* has not been investigated.

Treatment.—Considerable care is necessary in the treatment of enteric fever. The patient should not be permitted to leave his bed until convalescence has well advanced, should be fed on fluids only, and should be given no vegetable food. The diarrhœa should be carefully controlled, and constipation treated by enemata.

For tympanitis, peritonitis, &c., opium is the best remedy. Hæmorrhage should be treated with astringents and ice. Finally, it may be stated that antipyretic treatment, both by cold bathing and the administration of quinine, has proved very successful on the Continent and in England when it has been systematically carried out.

DIPHTHERIA.

Definition.—Diphtheria is an acute infectious disease in which there is a tendency to the formation of false membrane on mucous and abraded surfaces, chiefly of the fauces and respiratory tract, accompanied by considerable constitutional disturbance.

Symptoms.—After an incubation period, which varies greatly, but which is probably from twenty-four hours to ten days, shivering and vomiting set in, and the temperature becomes increased. The throat becomes sore, and there is some amount of stiffness about the neck. The fauces become of a dark red colour, the tonsils swollen, and at the end of two days from the beginning of the disease a quantity of minute white points appear on the surface of one or both sides of the

F

fauces. As these spots increase in number, they coalesce and form a thick yellowish white membrane. This sometimes consists of a single piece, but is often scattered over the surface in separate patches. The cervical glands become enlarged, the tongue coated with white or brown fur, the pulse and temperature increased, and the urine albuminous.

In the next stage the membrane separates, often leaving unhealthy sloughing ulcers.

In this stage recovery may take place, or death may result from exhaustion; during any period of the illness asphyxia, resulting from the production of false membrane in the larynx or bronchial tubes, may be fatal. In the course of the disease a roseolous rash may appear over the body. This is not different from the roseola which appears with other acute diseases.

Convalescence after diphtheria is very slow ; often paralysis of groups of the muscles shows itself within six months from the beginning of the attack.

Diagnosis.—Diphtheria may be confounded with (*a*) scarlatina, (*b*) tonsilitis, (*c*) herpetic sore throat. The points of difference between these diseases is shown in the following table :—

DIPHTHERIA.	SCARLATINA.
Throat of deep red, which is not uniformly distributed.	Throat of bright red, which is uniformly distributed.
Patches of thick yellow membrane on any portion of fauces.	Large white, thin, irregularly-shaped exudations on fauces.
Tonsils unequally swollen.	Both tonsils equally swollen.
Tongue coated with white fur.	Tongue furred, with large papillæ.

HERPETIC SORE THROAT.	TONSILITIS.
Throat less red than in scarlatina or diphtheria.	Throat less red than in scarlatina or diphtheria.
Small white points on tonsils.	Small thin, yellow exudation points over surface of tonsils.
Tonsils unequally swollen.	Tonsils unequally swollen.
Tongue furred.	Tongue furred.

Prognosis.—Diphtheria under any circumstances is a disease in which a guarded prognosis should be given. During the whole course of the disease symptoms may arise which are the precursors of a fatal termination.

Those cases are most serious which occur in young children, when there is a tendency to extension of the membrane, when an alteration in the voice betokens affection of the larynx, or when the powers of the patient begin to fail early.

Morbid Anatomy.—The diphtheritic poison, as it affects the mucous membrane, may give rise to two degrees of morbid changes—

1. The catarrhal stage, representing affection of the epithelial layers only, the disease not undergoing any further development.

2. The fibrinous stage, where, either with or soon after the catarrhal stage, there sets in an exudation of plasma, which gives rise to a fibrinous pseudo-membrane.

In the catarrhal stage, on making a section through the greyish white, slightly raised patch, the epithelial layer is not obviously thickened, and the greyish change extends only here and there into its substance. Numerous masses of micrococci are found on and in the superficial epithelial layers, forming somewhat flattened deposits. From these, processes of micrococci extend down into the rete Malpighii, spreading out here and there into roundish aggregations or colonies. The rete cells themselves are swollen, and have their nuclei more distinct.

Leucocytes next invade the diseased patch more and more, filling up all the space in the epithelium not already occupied by micrococci. Mingled with them there are large young cells, three or four times the size of leucocytes, and some multinuclear cells. This cellular or purulent infiltration helps to check the extension downward of the fungoid growth, and finally leads to the casting off of the patch of epithelium.

In the fibrinous stage, either soon after the appearance of the fungoid growth or after some pus formation, an exudation of plasma into the epithelial and subepithelial tissues lifts up the portion already infiltrated with micrococci, forming a thick false membrane, which soon undergoes necrosis. The surface consists of broken-down flakes and masses of epithelium, filled with micrococci, while in the deeper layers are loosened cells variously altered in shape and disintegrating, enclosed in a meshwork of fibrin filaments, with at first a few scattered leucocytes. Subsequent exudations of fibrin lift up the layers and thicken the fibres previously formed, giving the mass an amyloid appearance, and, on microscopic examination, the fibres are found to be fine in the subepithelial layers, becoming gradually coarser as the surface is approached. After twenty-four to forty-eight hours the rupture of the capillaries in the papillary layer gives rise to slight hæmorrhages, which are surrounded and shut off by subsequent fibrinous exudation. The cords of micrococci, extending gradually downwards towards the subepithelial layers, are thus being constantly pushed off towards the surface; but as the exudative process slackens, some of them extend into the lymphatic spaces of the tissue, filling them and the lymphatic vessels as well.

As the exudation of plasma finally ceases the purulent infiltration forms a line of demarcation, and with the increased secretion from the mucous glands either floats off the membrane *en masse* or checks the downward growth of the micrococci from the latter, which then slowly breaks down on the surface and is washed away.

Treatment.—The removal of the false membrane is of no avail; antiseptic applications are, however, very useful, and the patient's powers should be most carefully supported. The internal administration of the tincture of the perchloride of iron is valuable, both for its local action as an antiseptic and for its hæmatemic properties. If the larynx becomes affected, and there be much local obstruction to breathing, tracheotomy should be at once resorted to, for it is of no use to wait until the patient's powers are almost exhausted. The operation is itself a trivial one, and should therefore not be postponed.

CHAPTER VII.

Class I.—EXUDATIONES—*continued.*

Equinia—Pustula Maligna—Verruca Necrogenica—Frambœsia—
Erysipelas—Septicæmic Rashes—Surgical Rash.

EQUINIA—GLANDERS—FARCY.

Definition.—An acute infectious disease of the horse, ass, or mule, communicable to man by inoculation of a wound or abraded surface, and it is said by the prolonged contact of infected matter with the unbroken skin or mucous membranes, or by inhalation of air impregnated with the poisonous particles. It produces severe constitutional symptoms, and usually a pustular rash.

Symptoms.—The disease as it occurs in animals need not be discussed, except to remark that there is no essential difference between glanders and farcy. They are both caused by the same virus, both equally contagious, and differ only in certain clinical and anatomical details. The 'farcy buds' are merely one of the manifestations of 'glanders,' as a gumma or tubercular syphilide is of syphilis. According to the course and duration of the disease, an acute, subacute, and chronic form of glanders may be described. In acute glanders, after an incubation period of three to five days, or even of two or three weeks, *malaise*, loss of appetite, and obscure pains in the joints and muscles of the extremities are experienced. At the same time the skin round the wound or excoriation which has been inoculated becomes red, painful, and slimy; the lymphatics and glands become enlarged, red, and painful, and there is often an erysipelatous redness or cellulitis extending for a considerable distance round. The ulcer enlarges, its base and sides become corroded and greyish white with a foul discharge ; there is great prostration, with severe pain in the joints and muscles, and high fever is often present. Rigors are rare unless the disease is complicated with septicæmia.

If the attack be produced by inhalation of the poison, it commences with general symptoms only, and the first definite sign is the eruption. This consists of red spots—at first small papules, but soon enlarging into little indurated tubercles about the size of a pea—scattered over the face and more or less over the rest of the body. Pustules, and occasionally vesicles, soon form on their apices, burst, and leave foul ulcers. Sometimes larger nodules—farcy buds—at first form along the course of the lymphatics of the skin and subcutaneous tissue, but soon break down and suppurate, leaving deep irregular ulcers with sloughing surfaces. Similar nodules and abscesses in the intermuscular tissue, and suppuration in and around the joints, are often met with, also hæmorrhages into the swellings. In the affection of the mucous membranes, especially of the nose, either at the beginning, if the disease has been inoculated there, or after the previous phenomena, there is severe pain and swelling, with a mucous discharge, clear and viscid at first, but later brownish, offensive, and sanguineous. Tumours and ulcers may be found in the nose. Severe cough, pain in the chest, and expectoration of matter resembling the nasal discharge mark the implication of the lungs with the diseased growths. The pulse is small and frequent ; headache is often severe, and delirium is not uncommon.

In subacute glanders the symptoms are on the whole the same, only less intense and more protracted. The pain and the retarded suppuration caused by the ulcers usually produce a condition of hectic.

In chronic glanders there is, as in the acute forms, at first redness and swelling round the inoculated spot, with inflammation of the lymphatics, glandular enlargement, and some fever. The general symptoms subside for a time, but the ulcers go on slowly spreading in some places, healing in others. After a time nodular tumours or farcy buds, red spots, and pustules may arise, producing abscesses and ulcers on the skin, in the muscles, joints, and viscera. The nasal and other mucous membranes become affected, as in the acute form, and tubercles or ulcers about the larynx give rise to hoarseness or sudden œdema of the glottis. Bronchitis and pneumonia are frequently met with.

The fever may be high if there is much suppuration and rapid formation of abscesses, or may assume a hectic type.

Even in the event of a favourable course recovery is very slow, and often incomplete; the abscesses and ulcers gradually heal, the nasal discharge lessens and finally ceases, and the gastric and respiratory symptoms disappear. It is necessary to add that at any time the chronic variety may become acute and rapidly fatal.

Diagnosis.—The inoculation wound may be at first mistaken for the result of cadaveric poisoning, but is distinguished when the rash, nasal affection, and other symptoms set in. When acquired by inhalation, or where no wound is present, the early symptoms may lead to confusion with enteric fever if there is much pyrexia, *malaise*, headache, and delirium, or with rheumatic fever if the joint and muscular pains predominate. The appearance of the rash and nasal complication soon makes the diagnosis clear.

The papules may at first resemble those of variola, but they are larger and not 'shotty'; they soon develope into pustules and ulcers, instead of drying up into scabs; and abscesses, usually absent in variola, are almost constant in glanders.

Chronic glanders may be mistaken for syphilis; the history of contact with horses or persons suffering from the former, and the absence of the usual signs of the latter, will suffice to distinguish between the two diseases.

Prognosis.—Acute glanders is nearly always fatal, usually in seven or ten days from the onset of the attack. In the subacute forms of the disease death does not occur till after the second or third week, and about twenty-five per cent. recover.

In the chronic form the usual duration is about four months, and fifty per cent. recover.

Morbid Anatomy.—In acute glanders the cutaneous and nasal tubercles—farcy buds—so often met with in the horse, are frequently absent in man, and the morbid changes resemble those of pyæmia. As regards the skin, there are found, after death, scattered over the body, especially on the face and extremities, the red spots observable during life, with vesicles or pustules in some places and abscesses or ulcers in others. The vesicles containing caseo-purulent or bloody fluid have often a grey sloughy base. In the small cutaneous abscesses the pus is often of a viscid nature, and mixed with blood and shreds of tissue. Œdema, erysipelatous or phlegmonous changes, may also be present in the surrounding skin. The cutaneous nodules or tubercles are found to consist of localised deposits of small round cells in the sub-papillary layer of the corium, which at a later stage give rise to infiltration of the papillæ with leuco-cytes. The papillæ being thus disorganised, pus collects beneath the epidermis, forming a small abscess, which on burst-ing leaves a foul ulcer.

In the internal organs, such as in the mucous membranes of the nose, pharynx, and trachea, in the lungs, muscles, bones, and abdominal viscera, nodules, ulcers, abscesses, and hæmorrhages are frequently found.

Treatment.—No treatment is of any avail in the acute forms of the disease. In the chronic little can be done beyond keep-ing up the strength with a liberal and stimulating diet.

PUSTULA MALIGNA—MALIGNANT PUSTULE.

Definition.—A disease produced by the poison of animals suffering from charbon, characterised by the formation of a pustule, by subsequent gangrene, and by severe constitutional disturbance.

Symptoms.—It first appears as a small dark red patch, on which an elevation soon grows ; a small pustule forms on this and bursts. The inflamed area rapidly extends, becoming hard, and sloughs. Symptoms of severe constitutional disturbance accompany the local affection, and death frequently takes place in four or five days from the beginning of the disease. It is produced in man by direct contact with the diseased animal, but there is also some evidence that it can be conveyed by flies.

Diagnosis.—There is no disease for which malignant pustule can be mistaken.

Prognosis.—Usually fatal.

Morbid Anatomy.—Sections of the developing malignant pustule show that the central black spot is produced by hæmorrhage into tissue which has already undergone gangrene. There is acute inflammatory œdema around, and as the process of hæmorrhage and gangrene spreads gradually from the centre, we get finally the fully developed dark red or blackish spot covered with a vesicle containing blood-stained purulent fluid. The pustule is usually surrounded by extensive phlegmonous inflammation of the adjacent skin and subcutaneous tissue. The hæmorrhagic infiltration is seen to extend deeply into the substance of the corium, sending out reddish radiating branched processes. There is also more or less scattered hæmorrhage in the œdematous tissue, and in the corium in isolated patches. The fluid of the vesicle contains enormous quantities of slender, rod-shaped bacteria (*Bacillus anthracis*) aggregated in masses in the substance of the rete. As the disease advances they infiltrate the papillæ, hair follicles, sebaceous glands, and the deeper layers of the corium, finally making their way into the blood and infecting the body generally. An excess of leucocytes and plasma is present in the corium and papillæ. These bacilli have been cultivated out of the body, and after several generations had been obtained were found to produce anthrax when introduced into the bodies of animals.

Treatment.—In an early stage destruction of the affected part by caustics, or its entire removal by the knife, is advisable. If this be impossible, warm poultices should be applied, and attention should be directed to sustaining the patient's powers.

VERRUCA NECROGENICA.

Definition.—A disease occurring among those who are engaged as butchers or in making post-mortem examinations, and consisting of warts produced by infection from dead animal matter.

Symptoms.—The warts consist simply of patches of morbid growths, having somewhat the appearance of epithelial cancer.

Diagnosis.—The occupation of the patient readily enables the character of these growths to be recognised.

Prognosis.—They have a tendency to recur, but are otherwise innocent.

Treatment.—Removal by the knife or by caustics.

FRAMBŒSIA—YAWS.

Definition.—A contagious disease of the West Indies and Africa, rarely seen in this country, characterised by the appearance of a pustular eruption, which is replaced by a series of ulcers and attended by considerable constitutional disturbance.

Symptoms.—It commences with feverishness, and soon after small papules are produced, which are most numerous on the face and the extremities, and gradually grow until they reach the size of a sixpence. At the end of a few days a pustule forms on the elevation, and bursts, leaving a thick crust, beneath which ulceration takes place ; on this ulcer large granulations grow, giving an appearance which has been compared to a raspberry, but eventually these cicatrise and heal. This condition may go on for months, during which successive crops of the pustules may be produced. The constitutional symptoms are feverishness, sore throat, and sometimes dropsy.

Diagnosis.—There is no disease for which this can be mistaken.

Morbid Anatomy.—The morbid changes have not been investigated.

Treatment.—No specific treatment is known ; the ulcers

must be treated with stimulating applications, and the strength must be kept up with stimulants and a generous diet.

ERYSIPELAS.

Definition.—An acute contagious disease characterised by the production of a local inflammatory condition of the skin, and attended with symptoms of constitutional disturbance.

Symptoms.—There is still room for doubt whether an ordinary inflammation of the skin of itself can become erysipelatous, or whether a specific contagion is required for the production of the disease. It is certain, however, that wherever there is abrasion of the surface the skin at this point is likely to be attacked by erysipelas if the patient be exposed to unhealthy conditions—such, for instance, as a current of air escaping from a foul water-closet, or contact with decomposing matter. When once generated the inflammation spreads by extension to contiguous surfaces, and is easily conveyed by the hands of the attendants to other patients. It is the opinion of some that two forms of this disease exist—viz. a traumatic and an idiopathic erysipelas—and that the latter is not communicable. Evidence on this is, however, unsatisfactory; the belief probably arises from the fact that in hospitals the so-called idiopathic variety is usually treated in medical and not surgical wards, and that the patients therefore present no broken or absorbent surface for the reception of the poison.

The disease usually commences with a feeling of chilliness, headache, and often with vomiting. The tongue becomes furred, the pulse rapid, the temperature rises, and in severe cases the vomiting remains constant. There is a sensation of pain and itching at the seat of inflammation. When the part is first attacked the skin becomes red, shining, and slightly swollen, but the redness disappears temporarily on pressure. As the disease extends to the surrounding parts, the skin becomes of a darker red and the swelling increases, and at the end of about three days the redness may fade and the swelling subside, while the cuticle over the part desquamates.

In some cases the cuticle is raised into vesicles or bullæ, giving rise to the different varieties of erysipelas, to be described as follows :—

Erysipelas vesiculosum.—While the inflammatory condition exists a crop of small vesicles appears on the affected surface, which last a day or two, then burst and leave small brown scabs.

Erysipelas bullosum.—In this form, in which there is considerable swelling of the part after the inflammation has existed a few days, bullæ appear, which last a few days and then burst, leaving scabs.

Erysipelas pustulosum.—The contents of the vesicles or bullæ become purulent.

Erysipelas crustosum.—Simply a later stage of the former, characterised by the crusts which are formed (Hebra).

Erysipelas fugax.—The variety in which the inflammation moves from place to place, and is of short duration in each locality. In some cases the inflammation passes through some or even all the forms just mentioned above. In the majority of instances the area of redness is bounded by a well-defined line; but this is not always present, and it is sometimes difficult to determine the exact point where the inflammation ends and the healthy skin begins. The extent of surface covered is also very variable, being in some cases very limited, in others extending over the greater part or whole of the body, but the latter condition is very rare. The locality of the inflammation to some extent affects the course of the disease. Thus in *Erysipelas faciei* there is considerable œdema of the skin over the orbits, cheeks, and lips. This does not extend beyond the forehead, nor laterally beyond the ears; the rest of the surface is red but not swollen. The attack may be limited to one side of the face, but it usually extends to both, although its starting-point is on one side. It frequently arises from local breach of surface, due to some previously existing disease, such as otorrhœa, decayed tooth, or some skin eruption, such as eczema.

This variety is attended with considerable constitutional disturbance, often delirium. Other varieties of erysipelas are usually mentioned, being named after the parts of the body attacked; there is little to be said about them beyond the fact that the amount of swelling varies according to the denseness of the part. In those cases where the swelling is great, suppuration and sloughing often result, preceded by a dark purple appearance of the skin.

Diagnosis.—The local inflammation in erysipelas is distinguished from the more extended rashes of the acute specific diseases; from erythema it may be recognised by the absence of symptoms of constitutional disturbance, of swelling, and of desquamation in the latter, as well as by the rapidity with which the erythemata pass through their various stages.

Prognosis.—This depends upon the constitutional symptoms and the condition of health of the patient at the time when attacked. If the fever be high, if there be much delirium, if vomiting be constant, or if there be signs of exhaustion, the opinion must be guarded, as a fatal issue may occur rapidly. The facial variety is the most serious on account of brain complications. In the majority of cases recovery takes place.

Morbid Anatomy.—On cutting through the thickened and somewhat indurated portion of skin, the surface of the section shows the corium thickened, gelatinous-looking, and juicy, merging into the subcutaneous fatty tissue, with which it is in a manner blended. From the cut surface a sero-fibrinous fluid, containing leucocytes and a few red corpuscles, exudes.

Thin sections, under the microscope, show an abundant effusion of leucocytes throughout the whole of the affected tissue. The blood vessels especially are surrounded by thick cords of accumulated leucocytes, most marked in the marginal spreading part, where there are comparatively few connective-tissue spaces. Towards the centre the leucocytes are more diffusely spread, and are present in great numbers in and around the lymph spaces and lymphatic vessels. The endothelium of the latter is often swollen and granular, and sometimes is found desquamating. The epidermis, as well as the sweat and sebaceous glands and the hair follicles, becomes similarly affected with sero-fibrinous and cellular infiltration. The epidermic cells, especially those of the upper layer of the rete, are swollen, and as serum transudes it gradually separates the layers in the stratum lucidum and produces vesicles or bullæ. As the inflammatory process extends to the subdermic tissue, the fat cells, the blood and lymphatic vessels, become surrounded by lines of effused leucocytes. During the subsidence of the process the epidermis, owing to the alteration of the cells of the stratum lucidum having interfered with the conversion of their protoplasm into keratin, desquamates, and the degeneration and gradual absorption of the effused white and red corpuscles gives rise to a reddish brown stain.

Treatment.—At the onset of the attack a brisk purgative is necessary; and, indeed, during the whole course of the disease attention must be paid to the bowels. Iron in some form, and in large doses, is the most useful drug to be given. Locally the application of cold to the part is agreeable, and is probably of benefit; dusting with flour may be tried. Hebra recommends the application of mercurial ointment. Care should be taken to remove scabs retaining pus by means of poultices; suppuration should be treated with free incisions. It is believed by some that a superficial erysipelas in an early stage can be localised by drawing a ring round the affected part with a stick of caustic, but in practice this is often found to fail.

SEPTICÆMIC RASHES.

Definition.—Rashes occurring during septicæmia.

Symptoms.—During the septicæmic condition it is not uncommon to find rashes develope. They may appear as a simple hyperæmia, or consist of slightly raised patches or papules, which may be distinct from each other or may be confluent. The skin intervening between the papules may be normal in appearance or may be more or less injected. The papules, as a rule, fade on pressure, but return to their previous condition as soon as the finger is removed. Sometimes hæmorrhages take place from the edges of the papules, and give rise to a mottled appearance of the skin; these of course are not affected by pressure. In some cases, in addition to this rash, a quantity of vesicles or bullæ form; but these seem to be due to some neurotic condition, and more often follow an injury to the spinal cord. The papular rash usually first shows itself on the backs of the hands, wrists, the olecranon and patella; on the chest and abdomen the patches frequently are larger than on the extremities. The appearance of the rash is always, for a variable time, preceded by considerable constitutional disturbance, in nearly every case commencing with a severe rigor. The temperature is much increased, and the usual symptoms of septicæmia are present. These rashes may occur at any time when the patient is suffering from septicæmia.

Prognosis.—This is almost always unfavourable.

Treatment.—No local treatment is required.

SURGICAL RASH.

Occasionally, a few days after an operation, a roseolar rash appears over the body, attended with sore throat, high temperature, and other constitutional symptoms. Although mention of the affection has not been made under Scarlatina, there are many who believe it to be identical with this disease. The symptoms, it is true, have not been distinguished from those of scarlatina, to which it bears the closest resemblance, but sufficient evidence to prove their identity has not yet been adduced.

CHAPTER VIII.

Class I.—EXUDATIONES—*continued.*

SYPHILIS—INFANTILE SYPHILIS—VACCINO-SYPHILIS.

SYPHILIS—POX.

Definition.—A chronic infectious disease, produced by contagion or by inheritance from an affected parent, characterised by a train of definite symptoms, occurring in a definite order. According to Hutchinson it is a prolonged exanthem ; hence the position it occupies in this classification.

Symptoms.—Inoculation of the virus is followed by an interval during which no signs are manifested of its presence. This is the incubation period.

Occasionally a slight redness indicates some local irritation at the point where the poison was introduced, which, however, speedily subsides, and, unless the chancroidal virus has been mixed with that of syphilis, nothing as a rule is seen.

The primary sore makes its appearance between the fourteenth and thirtieth day after exposure to contagion. It is doubtful whether a shorter period than ten days ever elapsed between infection and development of the chancre ; on the other hand, it is unsafe to decide that syphilis has not been contracted because six weeks have not passed since the last known risk was incurred.

It is usual to divide the manifestations of syphilis into three classes or stages—primary, secondary, and tertiary.

The following table shows the period to which the chief symptoms and lesions are usually referred :—

PRIMARY.	SECONDARY.	TERTIARY.
Local Phenomena.	*Constitutional Phenomena.*	*Remote Phenomena.*
The chancre.	Induration of remote glands.	Arterial system: aneurism.
Induration of the chancre.	Pyrexia.	Nervous system: paralysis, &c.
Induration of near glands.	Sore throat.	Respiratory system:—
	Pain in limbs, &c.	Ulceration of larynx.
	Alopecia.	Phthisis.
	Iritis.	Osseous system:—
	Syphilides:—	Caries, &c.
	Roseola.	Liver ⎫
	Lichen.	Periosteum ⎪
	Psoriasis.	Testicle ⎬ Gummata
	Acne.	Cellular ⎪
	Vesicles.	tissue ⎭
	Condylomata.	Late syphilides:—
	Mucous tubercles.	Rupia.
		Impetigo.
		Ecthyma.
		Tubercles.
		Lupus.
		Ulcers.

Mr. Hutchinson has made the following convenient division of the course of the disease:—

A. *Incubation.*—From 'exposure' to induration of chancre and neighbouring glands; rarely less than ten days or more than six weeks; usually from three to five weeks.

B. *Development.*—From induration to appearance of rash, sore throat, and fever; two to four weeks.

C. *Exanthem Stage.*—So-called secondary symptoms. Very variable in extent, and dependent much on treatment; may exist for two years from infection, or even more.

D. *Post-exanthem Stage.*—A period of latency; sometimes with occasional relapses.

E. *Tertiary Stage.*—Period of 'remote sequelæ.' Symptoms proper to this stage rarely occur before six months from infection, or they may never manifest themselves at all. They may appear at any time throughout life, and are specially prone to do so when the patient is exposed to depressing influences, such as long, exhausting illness or privation.

The primary sore, or chancre—the initial lesion of syphilis —may present a great variety of appearances; it may exist by itself, or be complicated by the presence of a so-called 'soft chancre,' thus constituting a 'mixed' sore. It is rare to find more than one true chancre upon the same individual; yet exceptions to the rule are at times met with, notably in vaccino-syphilis. The seat of the sore is always at the point of inoculation; hence in the majority of cases it makes its appearance on some part of the genitals. It may, however, be accidentally produced on the finger, eyelid, tonsil, lip, tongue, navel, or anus. The most typical though by no means the most common form of primary sore is the 'true Hunterian chancre.' This commences as a small, almost painless papule, dusky red in colour, and slowly increases in size till it attains the proportions of a tubercle; when fully developed its dimensions vary from the size of a split pea to that of a sixpence; its outline, usually circular, may be modified by its situation: for instance, on the finger it may creep round the nail. After this, ulceration takes place upon the summit, with the formation of a greyish slough, often compared to moist wash-leather. The secretion is slight in amount, and consists of serum and epithelial débris, not of true pus. By the removal of successive sloughs the ulcer gradually deepens, and an excavated or crater-shaped depression is produced. Soon after the appearance of the chancre—generally within a week—a peculiar induration may be observed in the edges, base, and for a little distance in the surrounding tissues. It is of a tough consistency, much resembling cartilage and harder than ordinary inflammatory effusion, and is due to the presence of fibro-plastic elements, which infiltrate the layers of the corium and subcutaneous tissue. This condition, which to the touch feels like a coin or ring, may persist for some time after complete cicatrisation of the sore, but finally disappears by a process of fatty degeneration. It is most typical in parts where the connective tissue is abundant, such as the prepuce.

A far more common form of chancre is first noticed as a mere abrasion of the cuticle, which, instead of healing, increases in size, becomes slightly eroded, or in some cases elevated, is covered by a scanty, non-purulent secretion, undergoes induration, and finally heals with little or no contraction of tissue. In another variety a simple crack or fissure, which at first presents no appearance indicative of syphilis, obstinately refuses to heal, becomes indurated, and is followed by signs of constitutional infection. The amount of inflammation accompanying a primary sore varies much; it is generally slight, but when irritation is set up by caustics it may become excessive, and in delicate subjects may result in destructive phagedænic process. The duration of a primary sore is seldom less than two weeks and rarely more than three months.

Indolent enlargement of the glands nearest to the sore is usually observed within a week from the first appearance of the pimple or abrasion, but is attended with little or no pain. Suppuration occurs only in rare instances, where there has been much irritation of the primary sore.

Secondary Symptoms.—At a variable period after inoculation—generally between the eighth and eleventh week—signs of constitutional infection make their appearance. The primary sore by this time may have healed, but this is by no means the rule; and even in cases where the ulcer has disappeared the hard mass of induration will be easily felt. The first constitutional symptom is fever, which usually precedes the appearance of the rash on the body by twenty-four hours; it is not always well marked, and is said by Fournier to be more common in women than in men. In spite of the elevation of temperature there is, according to some, a craving appetite peculiar to this stage. The other symptoms are severe neuralgic headache, worse at night; great pain in the limbs, more especially

G 2

in the joints ; enlargement of the lymphatic glands throughout the system, particularly those of the occiput and axilla ; sore throat, and an eruption on the skin. The sore throat may commence as a simple erythema, but soon small shallow ulcers are seen scattered over the tonsils, root of the tongue, and upper part of the pharynx. Following the classification, and to a great extent the description, of Bäumler, we may divide the phenomena as seen on the skin into the following groups :—

I. Circumscribed hyperæmiæ with but slight infiltration—macular syphilide ; roseola.

II. Marked infiltration of the papillary body.

A. In the form of papules—papular syphilide.

B. In large patches—squamous syphilide.

On mucous membranes, or at favourable points on the cutis—moist papules (condylomata lata).

III. Especial implication of the immediate vicinity of the follicles (hair and sebaceous).

A. Simple infiltration with scanty or no exudation in the follicles—lichenous syphilide.

B. With acute suppuration in the follicle—acne syphilitica.

c. Exudation into small, markedly infiltrated groups of follicles with rapid formation of crusts—impetigo syphilitica.

IV. Infiltration with sub-epithelial suppuration and superficial ulceration—pustular syphilide (pemphigus syphiliticus, ecthyma syphiliticum, rupia syphilitica).

V. Infiltration with disintegration to a considerable depth (gummous)—tubercular syphilide.

Macular Syphilide—Roseola syphilitica.

This form of the exanthem is the first and most common. It consists of rose-coloured spots of a roundish or irregular shape, varying in size from a pin's head to that of a pea, disappearing on pressure and coming out in crops. The site varies with the severity of the attack. Sometimes but few spots are to be found on the chest, and in other cases the whole body may be covered. As a rule the eruption, if not treated, lasts for weeks, when it gradually fades, leaving slight coppery stains, which ultimately disappear. Occasionally roseola syphilitica relapses, when the spots differ somewhat from their original character, being paler in colour, fewer in number, and very often assuming an annular form.

Papular Syphilide.

When a case has been neglected this form of syphilide is often the first to appear, but it may be developed from the preceding variety. The papules vary in size from a grain of wheat to a pea, and are at first red in colour, gradually becoming darker. They are hard and usually smooth, but occasionally covered with small scales. The eruption may occur on any part of the skin, but its favourite sites are the borders of the scalp, the forehead—where it forms a band called the corona veneris—on the palms and soles, on the back of the neck, either in depressions or wrinkles, or on the flexor surfaces of the joints. If the papules are situated on the moister parts, such as the female genitals, or about the anus, or beneath the breasts, they may resemble the characters of condylomata. Relapses may take place late in the disease, when the papules are arranged in an annular form, often attacking unsymmetrically the palms and soles. The papules persist for a longer or shorter period, according to circumstances, and finally disappear, leaving a deeply pigmented stain.

Moist papules, or condylomata lata, are found on the mucous membranes as well as on the parts already mentioned, in the form of superficial white spots, in which there are abrasions of the membranes and a circumscribed thickening of the epithelium. They thus resemble the effect produced by nitrate of silver. The condylomata at times, and especially on the surface, will ulcerate, when the condylomatous ulcer is produced, but more frequently they spread rapidly, owing to the contagion of the secretion, and then appear in large masses.

Squamous Syphilide.

This form of syphilide arises either from a gradual enlargement of a single papule or from the coalescence of several papules, when the infiltration is excessive, causing desquamation on the surface. The appearance is somewhat that of common psoriasis, but the scabs are dirty in colour, quite different to the white transparent scales of the common disease. It may occur on any part of the body, but when, as is often the case, it appears late, it may show itself as a single patch of crescentic outline.

Lichen syphiliticus.

Occurs in the form of papules, which closely resemble simple milium, and consist of hard granules, like gum, found in the epidermis, which, when scooped out, leave small pits. They are at first red, but gradually become yellow, and are situated in groups of a dozen or more. When the inflammatory process that gives rise to them is severe, vesicles, or even pustules, may result.

Acne syphilitica.

In all respects, with perhaps the addition of a slightly coppery areola, this variety resembles acne vulgaris. The situation of the disease is the same in both, and the only point which can assist in the diagnosis is the presence of other syphilides on the skin. If the acne spots become pustular, with the rapid formation of crusts, syphilitic impetigo is produced.

Pemphigus syphiliticus.

Occasionally vesicles, large enough to deserve the title of bullæ, are seen, chiefly on the hands, and to them Bäumler has given this name. It is most common in hereditary syphilis.

Ecthyma syphiliticum.

Ecthyma is one of the later eruptions, occurring in the tertiary stage. It is unsymmetrical, altogether irregular, and characterised by pustules situated on inflamed bases. The pustules are caused by an infiltration into the epidermis of a fluid that rapidly becomes purulent. They soon burst, and so produce ulcers, which extend at the edges in a serpiginous manner, and when healed leave scars that may be pigmented.

Rupia.

This is the severest form of the pustular variety. It commences as a hard papule, which softens in the centre into a deep-seated pustule, which soon dries, and forms a conical-shaped scab, having the appearance of a limpet shell. When the scab falls off a foul circular ulcer is left, that ultimately cicatrises, leaving a permanent scar. It usually begins on the face, and extends to other parts of the body, chiefly the extremities. Rupia is generally unsymmetrical, and therefore a tertiary symptom, but in badly nourished persons it may occur comparatively early in the disease.

Tubercular Syphilide.

Tubercles are described as hard, flat, elevated bodies of a copper colour, which usually attack the face, tongue, penis, and limbs late in the disease. They commence as small papules, which enlarge and become scaly or scabby on the surface. Beneath the scales ulceration may take place.

Tertiary Symptoms.—Under the head of secondary symptoms all the syphilo-dermata have been briefly mentioned, it being impossible to divide them correctly into secondary and tertiary manifestations, because the numerous exceptions to the rule destroy the rule itself. The truth is, that all these varieties may occur more or less at the same time, or that they may overlap each other in such a way as to interfere with the conventional arrangement into fixed periods. Still it is useful, clinically, to retain the three divisions; and, more than that, there are certain general characters connected with the tertiary stage which help us to decide whether a symptom is a remote sequela or one of the acute phenomena of the disease.

Certain characteristics of the tertiary stage:—

1. Great obstinacy in healing and proneness to recur.
2. General absence of symmetry.
3. Invasion of deep organs and tissues as well as the superficial.

The late syphilides are most commonly of the pustular or tubercular type. The term syphilitic lupus is applied to a tubercular syphilide of the face, resulting in severe ulceration and extensive destruction of the bones and tissues; the name is ill-chosen, as it is apt to cause confusion with lupus vulgaris, which is not syphilitic. Ulcers are very common in this stage, and may arise as a result of boils, pustules, or tubercles. They are usually circular, with well-defined edges, looking as if they had been punched out with an instrument. They spread slowly, and destroy the deeper tissues in the process. A list of the other tertiary lesions has been given at the commencement of the chapter, and it is not within the scope of this work to do more than mention them.

Diagnosis.—The primary sore, or true chancre, has to be distinguished from the non-syphilitic chancre, or chancroid. The following are the chief points to be considered in deciding between them:—

1. *Site.*—It is extremely rare for the non-infecting sore to

exist upon any part except the genitals. The true chancre, though affecting the same locality, may be found elsewhere.

2. *Number.*—The soft sore has a tendency to multiplicity. The chancre, or hard sore, is usually solitary.

3. *Time of Appearance.*—The soft sore nearly always appears within three days of contagion. The hard rarely shows itself before the tenth day.

4. *Induration.*—Very slightly marked in a soft sore that has not been treated by caustics; well defined and cartilaginous in a chancre.

5. *Secretion.*—The soft sore secretes pure pus; the hard chancre, serum and epithelial débris.

6. *Bubo.*—The bubo resulting from a soft sore has a tendency to swell, be painful, and suppurate. The whole group of glands becomes glued together, and cannot be moved under the skin, whereas in the case of a true chancre the glands rarely suppurate unless the sore is irritated, or unless it takes on a phagedænic character. The ganglia become hard, are not glued together, remain freely movable under the skin, and are only slightly tender.

Herpes preputialis is sometimes mistaken for a chancre, but this mistake can only occur after the rupture of the vesicles, when the ulcer that is left resembles the 'simple abrasion' of primary syphilis. The history of a crop of vesicles, the smarting pain, the absence of induration, the date of appearance, and the rapid subsidence under simple treatment, are the main points to note in forming a diagnosis.

Syphilides, or Syphilo-dermata.

The general characteristics of skin eruptions due to syphilis are—

1. Tendency to present several types simultaneously. The macular, papular, and squamous forms constantly occur together, and may present every variety of intermediate stage.

2. A tint generally compared to 'copper' or 'raw ham,' and especially well marked in inveterate eruptions.

3. The general colour of the skin becomes yellow or earthy, implying the presence of a special cachexia.

4. Less itching than non-specific eruptions.

5. Tendency to leave brown stains, and to produce other pigmentary changes, such as leucoderma.

6. A disposition on the part of the ulcerative forms to spread in a characteristic serpiginous manner.

7. A tendency to attack the parts of the body not usually affected by the non-syphilitic eruptions, such as the flexor surfaces of the limbs, the palms, and soles.

Squamous syphilide, or syphilitic psoriasis, presents the following peculiarities :—

1. The production of scales is less profuse than in common psoriasis.

2. The white, glistening appearance of the patches is less marked, and there is a tendency to an ulcerative condition with the formation of dirty-coloured scabs.

3. The inner sides of the arms and thighs suffer more than the elbows and knees.

4. A decided tendency to affect palms and soles.

Syphilitic Iritis.—The lymph effused is seen in the form of patches or beads, especially at the margin of the iris, instead of appearing as a film covering the whole organ. There is also less pain than is the case with the traumatic and rheumatic varieties.

Syphilis of the Tongue, as a result of a gumma which has broken down, produces an obstinate, ragged ulcer, which has often the appearance of cancer. The history and the presence of other symptoms of syphilis will assist the diagnosis, while the scrapings, placed under the microscope, would indicate the presence or absence of the characteristic elements. Erichsen says, 'The syphilitic ulcer is elongated, irregular, and does not rapidly extend . . . . while the cancerous ulcer is of a more circular shape, has hard eroded edges, and spreads with greater rapidity.' Syphilis and cancer may both produce a hard, non-ulcerating tubercle in the tongue, but here, in addition to the history, we must bear in mind that cancer usually attacks the tip and edges, while syphilis affects the deep substance, of the organ. (Erichsen).

Prognosis.—The prognosis as regards absolute cure in a case of syphilis is most uncertain. It is true that many patients, after one or two attacks of secondary symptoms, if properly treated and of sound constitution in other respects, may never again be troubled by any manifestations of the disease. It is also, no doubt, true that the chance of immunity from fresh symptoms increases with the time that has elapsed since the disappearance of the last. Still, it is never safe to announce that we have seen the last of it. Any depressing influence, any severe illness, great privation, or over-work may excite the disease to renewed activity. Cases in which syphilis has reappeared after an apparent quiescence of twenty years are by no means rare. The important question, When may a man marry who has had syphilis? is one which ought to be considered under the head of prognosis. Much might be said upon the subject, but it will be sufficient here to assert that it is absolutely unsafe to marry until all constitutional signs of the disease have disappeared for at least twelve months. With the exception of infantile syphilis, which often destroys the child within a few months, it is only as a result of old-standing tertiary mischief that the disease is ever fatal.

Morbid Anatomy.—On examining under the microscope a *hard chancre* which has become fully developed, an infiltration of small round cells will be observed throughout the whole substance of the corium or mucous membrane, embedded in an amorphous or slightly granular substance, and specially numerous around the blood vessels, the walls of which are usually somewhat thickened and contain numerous round cells. As the cellular infiltration extends into the rete Malpighii, it produces impaired nutrition of the epidermis and subsequent scaling. In the later stages the conversion of the exuded cells into connective tissue maintains the induration, especially in the marginal part of the chancre.

The *roseolar syphilide* consists in a mere localised hyperæmia of the papillary layer, going on gradually to slight effusion of plasma, with accumulation of cells around the capillaries and a slight increase of nuclei in their walls.

In the *papular syphilide* the papillary layer is the seat of a cellular infiltration, identical in appearance with that of the hard chancre. The epidermis covering the little nodules becomes thinned or scaly, and occasionally a very slight subepithelial exudation gives rise to a shallow vesicle.

In ' *mucous tubercles* ' the same essential changes take place, but, under the influence of warmth and moisture, the papillary body hypertrophies, and the epidermis being macerated, a molecular ulceration of the exposed papillæ occurs. 'Mucous tubercles' that are kept dry assume the appearance of ordinary papular syphilides.

The *squamous syphilide*, due to the enlargement of a syphilitic papule or to the coalescence of several, presents similar anatomical changes.

In the simplest cases of *lichenous syphilide* there is an infiltration of small round cells just outside the hair and sebaceous follicles, combined with hyperæmia of the follicular plexus. In more acute cases there is slight exudation into the follicles, forming minute discrete vesico-pustules, which soon dry up and, falling off, leave small dark, depressed, slowly-fading scars.

Occasionally the intervening skin between the papules becomes affected, and the papillary layer being infiltrated, the little group of lichenous spots becomes converted into a scaly eruption.

If the process be still more acute, leading to suppuration in and round the follicles, the *acneiform syphilide* is produced ;

and if the skin intervening between the follicles becomes affected, an aggregation of closely-packed pustules on an inflamed base is formed, which soon becomes covered with a greenish-yellow granular crust, producing the *impetiginous syphilide*.

In the *vesicular* and *bullous syphilides* the serous effusion into the epidermis, separating the cells of the stratum lucidum, gives rise to vesicles, the contents of which, often turbid and blood-stained from the first, soon become purulent. The crusts formed by the drying up of the contents leave only a slight scar on falling off. If the base of the vesicle becomes red and inflamed, and the rete with the papillary layer be more or less destroyed, the so-called *ecthymatous syphilide* is produced. Owing to the loss of time, the scars left after separation of the scabs and healing of the ulcers are depressed, and often deeply pigmented.

By an extension of the infiltration round the periphery of the scab, successive layers are added from below, and a conical prominence, seated on a purplish-red ulcerated surface, is gradually formed, termed the *rupial syphilide*.

In the *tubercular syphilides* there is a formation of gummata in the substance of the true skin. In the deeper layers of the corium there are seen small nodules, greyish red and homogeneous on section, and merging gradually into the surrounding tissue, so that they cannot be enucleated.

Microscopically they consist of masses of round cells closely aggregated together in a meshwork of fine fibres. The marginal portions in older nodules, and the whole mass in the younger ones, are pretty freely supplied with vessels ; but in process of growth these get gradually obliterated in the centre, which then undergoes mucous or caseous degeneration. The margin, qn the other hand, may undergo condensation from partial conversion of the round cells into spindle cells and connective tissue. As the nodule extends towards the surface, the swelling, which at first has presented the appearance of a colourless papule, becomes redder, and, slowly involving the papillary layer, causes irritative changes in the epidermis. These may result in desquamation only, or, by the exudation of a little serum, in the formation of a thin yellowish crust. Sometimes, also, a vesicle is formed, which dries up to produce a crust, beneath which ulceration of the tubercle slowly takes place. If the tubercle be large and softened in the centre, when it reaches the skin a bluish-grey furuncle-like body is formed, which on bursting discharges a yellowish material, and in consequence a deep, slowly-spreading ulcer is produced.

Infantile or Inherited Syphilis.

A child may inherit syphilis from either parent, but in the majority of cases the mischief may be traced to the father. This arises from the fact that a woman whose constitution is infected at the time of conception, or becomes so during gestation, is particularly liable to abort. When delivery takes place at full term, the child rarely survives it more than a few·weeks. It should be mentioned here that some deny the possibility of direct contamination of the fœtus by the father, and maintain that the mother is always intermediately infected. Nothing is known with certainty of the means by which the disease is transmitted, but it is certain that the placenta not uncommonly shows traces of the malady. (Virchow).

Infantile syphilis may either appear at or soon after birth, or may not give any signs of its presence till several weeks have elapsed. The former cases are the more serious, and usually terminate fatally. They are characterised by a bullous or pustular eruption, which never appears later than the first week. The first seat is generally on the palms and soles, spreading thence to the trunk, limbs, and occasionally to the face. Dirty red, circular spots, of variable size, are first seen, and effusion beneath the cuticle converts these into blebs, which after a time rupture and produce unhealthy excoriations, obstinately resisting treatment. Fresh crops of blebs appear, some of which at times attack the mouth and nose. The nails fall off, and finally the child becomes a mass of ulcerating sores, and succumbs in less than a month. The name pemphigus neonatorum was applied to this form of the disease before its nature was understood, but it is more correct to call it pemphigus syphiliticus.

In the more numerous class of cases the child may be apparently healthy at birth, or merely somewhat undersized. After a period, varying from a fortnight to two months, it becomes emaciated, delicate, and irritable; the skin is shrivelled, rough, dry, and of a peculiar earthy colour. Mucous tubercles, accompanied by catarrh of the nasal mucous membrane, make their appearance, and give rise to much swelling and profuse thin secretion. The characteristic noise produced by the child's efforts to remove the obstacle to respiration has obtained for this symptom the name of '*the snuffles.*' At about the same time as the coryza an eruption appears, usually commencing about the anus and buttocks, whence it may extend to any or every part of the surface, more especially over the face. Macules, papules, and scaly patches, in varying proportions, make up a rash of a mixed character, which it is impossible to refer to any one form. The colour, however, presents the copper tint of syphilis.

Condylomata about the anus cause much trouble, and ' rhagades' are found in that situation, and about the mouth, where they leave scars.

In addition to these symptoms the infant usually suffers from severe diarrhœa, stomatitis, and loss of flesh and hair, and in consequence assumes the aspect of an old man. At the end of twelve months, if properly treated, all these symptoms subside. Tertiary manifestations make their appearance between the ages of four and fourteen. As in the adult, they appear in the bones and deeper tissues as well as in certain eruptions, such as rupia and ecthyma. Besides these there are certain lesions which are specially characteristic of the inherited form of the disease.

A. Cloudiness and opacity of the cornea, known as 'interstitial keratitis.'

B. Certain changes in the teeth, probably the result of early stomatitis. These changes are most marked in the permanent set, but may be observed to a less extent in the milk teeth. The incisors, especially those of the upper jaw, suffer most, the median being first attacked. They are small in size and pegged, rapidly wear away, and present a notch in the centre of the edge and a wide interval between them. The canines suffer, but to a less extent. (Hutchinson).

C. Depression of the nasal cartilages produces the remarkable flattening of the bridge of the nose.

D. Less common than any of the preceding is an enlargement of the lower end of the humerus and sternal end of the clavicle.

Vaccino-Syphilis.

The series of carefully observed cases reported by Mr. Hutchinson in this country, and the report by Dr. Pacchiotti, of Turin, who was specially employed to observe an outbreak of the disease in the Rivalta valley in 1861, leave no doubt that syphilis is occasionally produced in healthy persons by careless vaccination with lymph taken from infected children. Under these circumstances the disease runs precisely the same course and exhibits the same symptoms as when inoculation takes place in other ways.

Treatment.

Primary Sore.—There is considerable doubt whether any good is gained by the vigorous cauterisation of the primary sore, which is so strongly recommended by some surgeons; at all events, if the plan is adopted, it must be done early and with the strongest form of caustic, such as pure nitric acid. The usual and best local application is black wash. When a case is decided to be one of syphilis, no time should be lost in giving the antidote, which is undoubtedly mercury. Some authorities recommend waiting till the secondary symptoms have shown themselves before using the remedy, but it is better to try and lessen their severity by its early use.

In administering the drug we may select from a large number of methods, of which the following are the most important :—

A. *By the Mouth.*—One drachm of the solution of corrosive sublimate three times a day; four or five grains of blue pill, with a little opium, night and morning; one grain of the green iodide three times a day, or five grains of Plummer's pill as often, are the best preparations to be used.

B. *By the Rectum.*—Bryant advises the use of mercurial suppositories.

C. *By Hypodermic Injection.*—Four grains of the perchloride in an ounce of water; fifteen minims for a dose.

D. *By Vapour Baths,* using from ten to thirty grains of calomel for each bath.

E. *By Inunction.*—A drachm of mercurial ointment may be rubbed into the axillæ or groins night and morning.

Two or more of the preceding modes may be used together, and it is sometimes an advantage to vary during the treatment the mode of administering the drug. In a mercurial course attention should be paid to the following points :—

1. Avoid profuse salivation. The gums must be carefully watched, the teeth being cleansed twice or three times daily with an aromatic or astringent wash.

2. Warn the patient against catching cold.

3. Continue the treatment for some time after the disappearance of the symptoms, and discontinue the use of the drug gradually rather than suddenly.

4. Give a simple and nutritious diet, with a moderate amount of good wine and beer. Avoid fruits of all kinds.

H

5. Stop the use of the drug, or give it very cautiously, if the patient is cachectic, and substitute for it iron, cod-liver oil, and other tonics.

Secondary Symptoms.—They should be treated on a similar plan—that is, by the administration of mercury, if it has not been already commenced during the primary stage. Ulcers in the mouth and throat should be lightly touched with nitrate of silver or with a solution of perchloride of mercury.

Condylomata about the anus, &c., are best treated by dusting them with calomel.

Tertiary Symptoms.—Mercury by the mouth, with only a few exceptions, should be avoided in this stage, especially when the deeper tissues are involved. In its place the drug to be relied upon is iodide of potassium, which should be given in full doses of ten to thirty grains three times a day.

Gummatous deposits in the skin should be treated locally, by means of mercury ointment, or the oleate of mercury. In this stage good food, wine, change of air, and general tonics are of great importance.

Infantile syphilis must be treated by mercury. The usual modes of administering it are by the mouth, in the form of one or two grains of grey powder, night and morning, or by the inunction of mercurial ointment, which is most easily applied on the child's abdominal binder.

CHAPTER IX.

*Class I.—*EXUDATIONES*—continued.*

Sub-class B.—*Of Internal or Local Origin.*

1. *ERYTHEMATOUS GROUP.*

Erythema simplex, læve, fugax, intertrigo; multiforme, including papulatum, tuberculatum; annulare, iris, gyratum—Erythema nodosum—Roseola—Urticaria—Pellagra.

ERYTHEMATA.

Definition.—The erythemata are characterised by the existence on the skin of dusky red, slightly raised patches of various sizes, which occasionally vesicate, run an acute course, and are attended with little or no constitutional disturbance.

Symptoms.—When the patches first appear, they are surrounded by a hyperæmic zone, which prevents their margin being clearly defined; at the end of a few hours this zone disappears without leaving any pigment, and the erythematous papules can be distinctly recognised. After lasting a few days the papules fade, and are usually followed by desquamation, which is limited to the site of the eruption. In some cases, during the height of eruption, a small vesicle or bulla may be produced. There is no itching, and but little, if any, constitutional disturbance. The papules are most frequently found on the back of the hands and the dorsum of the feet, where, as a rule, they commence even when they extend to other parts of the body. They occur less often on the arms and legs, and seldom extend to the face and trunk of the body, never without implicating the limbs. A large number of varieties of this rash

H 2

have been described by different writers, depending on differences noticeable in the character of the eruption itself, in its
site, and in the amount of constitutional disturbance it produces.

With one exception, to be afterwards mentioned, they are
attended by but little if any increase of temperature; indeed,
but for the appearance of the rash there is nothing in the
patient's condition, either local or constitutional, which would
attract attention to the disease. They all agree in the rash
being unilateral; when the trunk is implicated, both sides of
the body are affected at the same time. The duration of the
disease varies greatly, and it often has a tendency to return to
parts which have been attacked in the first instance, and from
which the eruption has already faded.

Erythema læve occurs as the result of venous obstruction,
and is a mere hyperæmia of the skin; it frequently is a consequence of some general condition, such as dropsy, and is more
often seen on the legs. The redness is preceded by œdema of
the skin, and may not progress further than the stage of hyperæmia, but occasionally bullæ form on the surface.

Erythema fugax is a simple hyperæmia of the skin, which
is due to gastric disturbance or local irritation. It consists of
patches of redness of irregular shape, which appear in different
parts of the body, frequently on the face and upper part of the
trunk. The patches are of very short duration, come and go
rapidly, and in most cases itch and tingle while present.

Although these diseases are usually described as erythemata, it is doubtful whether they should not, as Hebra suggests, be excluded on the ground that they are only hyperæmiæ
of the skin.

Erythema intertrigo is a local erythema, produced by the
friction of opposed surfaces of the skin, and occurs in fat persons, more particularly children. It soon becomes moist, when
it assumes the nature of an eczema, under which head it will be
again noticed.

Of the other varieties described by different writers, such as

Wilson, Rayer, and Fuchs, only those included by Hebra under the name of erythema multiforme will be noticed. Hebra looks upon these varieties as merely different stages of development of the same eruption; thus E. papulatum and E. tuberculatum differ from each other simply in the size of the patch, in the former being about the size of a pin's head or larger, in the latter about the size of a fourpenny piece. They occur generally on the backs of the hands and feet, and occasionally extend to the arms and legs, and rarely to the face and body. In both forms they are of a dusky red or violet colour, and when they first make their appearance are surrounded by a zone of redness, which lasts but a few hours. At the end of three or four days they fade, occasionally leaving a temporary yellow stain, due to escape of colouring matter of the blood into the skin. A slight desquamation follows the fading of the papules. The papules are succeeded by others, but the whole course of the eruption is limited to a few days. The young are most frequently affected by this form of erythema, most often in the spring and autumn of the year. A difference of opinion exists as to which sex is most frequently attacked.

Erythema annulare results when the erythematous patch begins to fade in its centre, leaving a red ring surrounding a pale surface.

Erythema iris is produced when a second or third ring is formed outside the inner, due to a fading of the redness in the circumference of the patch. In this, as in all varieties, vesication may take place.

Erythema gyratum is said to occur when portions of the rings of E. iris fade, and in consequence of several patches being close the rings run together, forming a serpentine eruption.

The circular form of erythema differs only from the papular in the appearance of the eruption. They present themselves on the same parts of the body, last but a few days—never beyond a month—and cause almost no constitutional disturbance.

ERYTHEMA NODOSUM.

This variety of erythema differs widely from the preceding forms in the character of the eruption—in its site, in its symptoms—and, in fact, it is not a skin disease at all. It consists of oval swellings, at first hard, but at a later stage soft, from a half to four or five inches in length. At the commencement the swellings are pale red, but gradually become of a dark red or violet colour. After a few days, as the colour fades, it is replaced by a yellow discoloration, which persists for some time after the disappearance of the swelling. These swellings occur in crops of rarely less than a dozen in number, most frequently on the front of the lower extremities, but are by no means limited to this site. A second, sometimes even a third, crop makes its appearance, invading parts which in the first attack have escaped, and thus the eruption extends over other parts of the body. This form of erythema is not attended by any itching, but is characterised by considerable pain at the seat of eruption, and great general debility, anæmia, and gastric disturbance.

Diagnosis.—Simple erythema can only be confounded with prurigo, from which, however, it can be distinguished by the extreme itching and blood crusts of the latter, and by the limitation of the rash of prurigo to the back and extensor surfaces of the arms and legs; while erythema attacks the anterior surface as well. The varieties of erythema multiforme can hardly be mistaken for any other disease, with the exception, perhaps, of the gyrate form, which may be taken for ringworm of the body. The rapidity of the appearance and disappearance of the former, and the absence of microscopical evidence, are points to guide us in our diagnosis.

Erythema nodosum can be readily distinguished from all other eruptions by the tenderness of the patches, the pain they occasion, and by the constitutional and gastric symptoms which accompany it, as well as by the gradual alteration in colour from day to day, resembling a bruise.

Prognosis.—Always favourable, although the period of duration varies. Death after E. læve results not from the erythema, but from the disease during which it occurs. The length of an attack of E. nodosum depends on the number of crops which appear; five or six weeks is, however, an outside limit. Like the rest of the erythemata, the symptoms disappear spontaneously.

Morbid Anatomy.—The changes in the skin may be due to—

1. Simple hyperæmia of the superficial layer of the cutis.
2. Hyperæmia followed by exudation.

The former exists in E. simplex and in E. intertrigo.

On examining the affected portion of the skin with a simple lens, magnifying about twenty diameters, a great number of minute red dots are seen, which are the tops of the capillary loops in the papillæ, especially in the region of the hair follicles. As the turgescence of the minute vessels passes off readily, no morbid appearances are to be found after death.

In the latter condition, in addition to the simple hyperæmia of the papillary layer, there is exudation of plasma, of pale and then of red corpuscles, according to the severity of the process, followed often by various secondary inflammatory changes. In E. papulatum, following on the hyperæmia, there is slight effusion of plasma in the substance of the papillary layer, giving rise to slight elevation of the little spots. An excess of serum, transuding into the epidermis, and collecting in the stratum lucidum, may give rise to minute vesicles. In E. nodosum a number of pale, together with a few red, corpuscles, as well as a large amount of plasma, are effused. The exudation pressing on the vessels, gives rise, as in a wheal, to the pallor in the centre of the patch, and the breaking-down and pigmentary changes in the red corpuscles produce the purplish, greenish, and yellow discoloration in the same way as in a fading bruise.

Treatment.—In the treatment of E. læve every care should be taken to assist the circulation of the part ; the limb should be raised, carefully supported, and warm fomentations applied.

Often acupuncture by means of Southey's trocars becomes necessary to relieve the œdema. Bathing the part with an astringent lotion is recommended.

In E. fugax the diet should be carefully regulated. Often this eruption is due to the use of soap, which should of course be avoided. Local treatment is unnecessary, not only in this form but in all the varieties of erythema, on account of the short duration of the eruption. In E. intertrigo attention should be paid to keeping the part dry and clean; a weak tar lotion is of use. The constitutional treatment of all the erythemata should consist in regulating the bowels and in the subsequent administration of acid and bitter tonics.

ROSEOLA.

Much difference of opinion exists among dermatologists concerning the diseases usually classed under this heading. Willan has described, under the name of roseola, a variety of rashes which are not recognised by all writers, and Hebra especially doubts their existence. There may be some difficulty in agreeing with Willan in the correctness of describing as separate affections R. infantilis, R. æstiva, R. autumnalis, R. annulata, but we shall mention a rash under the name of roseola which is by no means limited to one period of the year. A roseolous rash, occurring in association with some of the acute infectious diseases, has been described under the head of these diseases.

Definition.—Roseola is an acute disease characterised by the production on the body of small rose-coloured papules, and attended by very slight constitutional symptoms, which make their appearance at the same time as the rash.

Symptoms.—The rash consists of minute red and slightly elevated spots, scattered over the chest and neck, less often extending over the face and arms. They disappear temporarily on pressure, last but a few days, and fade, leaving a discoloration of the skin, but are sometimes followed by slight desquamation. Feverishness, headache, and occasionally vomiting are present at the commencement of the rash.

The constitutional symptoms are, however, slight; the temperature is seldom as high as 102° Fahr., and more often only just above normal. The fauces are frequently a little injected, but the redness does not extend beyond the edge of the soft palate, and the tonsils are not swollen. The tongue is slightly furred, and the papillæ along its edge are often prominent.

Diagnosis.—Roseola is often mistaken for scarlatina, and the diagnosis between the two affections is frequently a matter of considerable difficulty. They differ in the fact that the papules in the former are more widely separated from each other than those in the latter, and the skin intervening between the papules does not become red in roseola, as it does in scarlatina. The constitutional symptoms in roseola appear at the same time as the rash, while in scarlatina they precede it. Roseola is not infectious, and occurs more frequently among young women and children than other persons. Also see table, pp. 43, 44.

Prognosis.—Roseola always ends in recovery in a few days.

Morbid Anatomy.—The changes are the same as in the milder forms of erythema, the processes usually stopping short at hyperæmia only, but sometimes going on to slight exudation of plasma. The vascular plexuses round the hair follicles, sweat and sebaceous glands, are the regions specially involved.

Treatment.—Nothing is required beyond rest for a day or two.

URTICARIA—NETTLE RASH.

Definition.—A disease the chief symptom of which is the production of wheals on the skin, causing great irritation, usually unattended by any constitutional symptoms, but sometimes by fever, pain in the epigastrium, and headache.

Symptoms.—The eruption makes its appearance at the same time as any constitutional symptoms which exist, and consists of a quantity of wheals. These vary greatly in size, in quantity, in shape, and in colour; but the difference in the variation in colour is due to their being in different stages of development. As a rule they appear first as red elevations, which increase in size, becoming white in the centre with red margins. They may occur on any part of the body, and although each individual wheal does not last many hours, a succession may make their appearance for weeks or months. They are accompanied by a severe itching or stinging sensation of the part, and constitutional symptoms may or may not be present.

In some individuals a condition of skin exists which may fairly be considered to result from an urticarial diathesis.

Several forms of urticaria are recognised.

Urticaria febrilis.—In this form the eruption is preceded by shivering, headache, furred tongue, and vomiting. Soon a number of slightly raised wheals appear over the greater proportion of the body, and usually begin on the wrists and neck. These come and go rapidly, and the itching is intolerable, so much so that it is impossible not to rub or scratch them. Wherever the skin is touched fresh wheals appear, till in this way the surface is more or less covered. From the scratching the skin becomes excoriated, but desquamation does not occur at any time. The irritation is always worse at night.

Urticaria conferta is a chronic variety of the disease in which the wheals are abundant but limited to one or two localities.

Urticaria evanida is also a chronic form, in which the wheals come and go rapidly.

Urticaria perstans is a variety in which the eruption continues without changing for some weeks, and may perhaps be the same form which has been well called by Dr. Alfred Sangster Urticaria pigmentosa, in which the wheals last for years, leaving a deposit of pigment, which causes a mottled appearance on the skin.

Urticaria tuberosa is rarely seen; in it the wheals are of a larger size than in the others, and it occurs in persons of weak constitution.

Urticaria miliaris, U. vesicularis, U. bullosa, are described and so called because vesicles or bullæ form on the surface of the wheal. They are extremely rare.

In *Urticaria papulosa* the wheals are so small as to resemble papules. Hebra says that they increase in size, but later in the disease diminish again.

Diagnosis.—Urticaria is easily distinguished from the erythemata by the more diffused character of the eruption and the difference in the site, by the absence of local irritation in erythema, by the urticarial wheals being white in the centre with red margins, and more raised than the erythematous patches; from measles and scarlatina by the absence of coryza and sore throat in urticaria, and its lowness of temperature, and by the different courses these diseases run; from erythema nodosum by the presence of itching in urticaria and heat and pain in the former.

The ease by which the rash is excited in certain varieties of urticaria by the slightest irritation of the skin is often a useful diagnostic sign.

Urticaria often arises from the ingestion of some special article of food, such as mussels, oysters, cucumber, mushrooms, &c., and even cold water; but in many persons it arises without any apparent cause. It is undoubtedly affected by season, in some being worse in cold than in hot weather. The young are more liable to it than the old, and it is occasionally associated with irregularities of menstruation, pregnancy, the presence of parasites in the alimentary canal, and arises very frequently from the irritation caused by the bites of fleas, bugs, &c.

Prognosis.—Urticaria is not a fatal disease. As a rule an attack passes off in a few days, but it may be extremely obstinate and resist all forms of treatment.

Morbid Anatomy.—On examining a vertical section of an urticarial wheal we find the connective-tissue bundles of the corium separated by effused plasma. The capillaries and small vessels are dilated, especially in the marginal zone of the wheal, full of blood, and surrounded by lines of effused leucocytes, which are present in larger numbers than normal throughout the whole corium. The lymphatics of the skin are widely dilated and full of lymph. In some cases escape of red corpuscles by transudation, or actual rupture of the vessels, gives rise to pigmentary and other colour changes in the wheal.

Each wheal usually corresponds with the area of distribution of a terminal arteriole, and is supposed to be produced by paralysis of the vasomotor nerves supplying the branch; but opinions differ as to the way in which this can give rise to exudation.

Treatment.—If a cause, either internal or external, can be found for its existence, it should be at once removed.

In acute urticaria it is well to begin with an emetic or purgative, or both. In both acute and chronic forms it is important to diet the patient carefully, paying particular attention to avoid his having indigestible food, salt meat, pork, &c. The bowels should be regulated, and the patient kept cool. With a view to allay irritation, sponging the skin with cold water should be adopted. Saline baths and lotions are useless, but washing with weak vinegar is agreeable, and should be persisted in if the irritation be severe. Aconite has been given internally with doubtful benefit, but arsenic is certainly of value in some of the more persistent forms of the disease.

PELLAGRA—ITALIAN LEPROSY.

Definition.—Pellagra is a serious disease, occurring endemically in Northern Italy and Southern France, one of its chief characteristics being an erythema of the skin. This appears on those parts of the body most exposed to the sun, such as the hands and arms, neck and chest. Women suffer from it on the face, owing to the fact that their head dresses do not protect them from the sun's rays, while among men, whose faces are screened by large hats, this part is more rarely affected.

Symptoms.—It commences as a mere erythema of the skin, which is accompanied by a sense of irritation. During the winter this subsides, but a deposit of more or less pigment remains. Vesication does not occur, but the erythema is followed by desquamation. On the return of the summer the erythema again makes its appearance, and each year the skin is left more stained with pigment. At first the patient simply complains of lassitude, but gradually becomes melancholic; later on suffers from marked cerebral symptoms, which terminate in insanity.

Prognosis.—The length of the disease—that is, from first symptom to death—varies from a few to ten or twelve years, usually about five. Although it generally proves fatal, this is not always the case; but even when recovery takes place it is only partial. Complete restoration to health is rare.

The causes of pellagra are not well understood. It is a disease altogether confined to the poor, and to those who work in the sun. It has been attributed to the character of the food which these people eat, and has been thought to be associated with maize, their chief article of diet. In the damp seasons maize is attacked with a parasitic fungus, which is supposed by Bellardine to be the origin of pellagra. When maize is supplemented by other food, as in the large towns, the disease does not exist. Pellagra is not contagious, nor is there any evidence that it is hereditary, although members of the same family who are exposed to the same conditions are often attacked with it together.

Treatment.—The treatment of the local inflammation is simple. Protection from the rays of the sun always leads to a subsidence of the symptoms. As has been explained, a nourishing and varied diet in the early stages of the disease will often restore the patient to health.

CHAPTER X.

Class I.—Exudationes—*continued.*

2. *PAPULAR GROUP.*

Lichen simplex, ruber, planus, marginatus, scrofulosorum—Prurigo
—Prurigo Infantum—Relapsing Prurigo.

Lichen.

Under the title of lichen a considerable number of diseases
have been described, many of them presenting appearances
which differ very widely from each other. Willan includes not
only those conditions which will shortly be described, but
others which differ in their course as well as in their appearance; thus 'Lichen pilaris' of Willan is more fitly described as
a disease of the hair follicles, and is apparently the disease which
Devergie called Pityriasis pilaris, while the Lichen agrius and
Lichen tropicus of Willan are believed by Hebra to be varieties
of eczema. Hebra, indeed, objects to Willan's Lichen simplex,
on the ground that it is an acute disease of the skin, but in the
following account L. simplex will be retained for the reason
that, with this exception, its appearance and course are such as
necessitate its association with the other forms which are
accepted by Hebra as true lichens. We shall therefore limit
ourselves to describing three forms—L. simplex, L. ruber of
Hebra or L. planus of Wilson, and L. marginatus, including
scrofulosorum.

Definition.—Lichen may be defined as a papular disease of
the skin, with more or less local irritation.

LICHEN SIMPLEX.

Lichen simplex is characterised by a group of minute papules, that appear more frequently on the back of the neck and upper extremities, but often on other parts of the body. The papules are acuminated and of a red colour, and last a variable time, usually about five or six days. They gradually disappear, and are followed by trifling desquamation. Occasionally slight signs of constitutional disturbance accompany the local symptoms, such as feverishness and headache. Locally an itching or tingling sensation is present at the site of the eruption.

LICHEN RUBER (*Hebra*), LICHEN PLANUS (*Wilson*), LICHEN PSORIASIS (*Hutchinson*).

Lichen ruber of Hebra is comparatively rare in this country. Hebra describes it as ' an eruption of miliary papules which are at first distinct from one another, and covered with thin scales.' The papules remain the same size during the whole course of the disease. Successive crops of the eruption appear, and thus the papules become aggregated together; eventually they are so closely placed that they come in contact with each other, and in this way are formed 'continuous patches of variable size and shape, red, infiltrated, and covered with scales.' As the disease progresses the patches extend over different parts of the body, the skin becomes greatly thickened, and when this condition exists over joints their movement is interfered with. Frequently in the folds of the skin over the joints of the fingers fissures occur and extend into the corium, becoming filled with black crusts of blood. The natural lines and wrinkles about the face disappear, the nails become either greatly thickened, brittle, and of a yellowish brown, or thin and of a light colour. The hair of the head, pubes, and axillæ is never affected. This variety itches but little.

Under the names of Lichen planus and Lichen Psoriasis

Wilson and Hutchinson describe diseases which are probably the same as the Lichen ruber of Hebra. Mr. Hutchinson, in his 'Lectures on Clinical Surgery,' 1879, says, ' Under slightly different names Hebra and Wilson have independently described this disease, and have agreed most closely as to all its main features.'

This disease usually presents itself in the form of patches of a round or oval shape, or running in lines, and consists of an aggregation of small round flat-topped papules, some of which may have a minute central depression, which is the opening of a hair follicle. In the earlier stages of the disease the papules are more scattered, but as the eruption developes they increase in number, and have a tendency to become confluent, often forming patches resembling common psoriasis; this, however, never results from the increase in size of the individual papules. The papules are of a livid red, or violet tint, and each is covered with a small thin scale. Often the eruption has at first sight an appearance like herpes, which on closer observation is found to be due to the shiny character of the scales. The patches never are moist, and have no tendency to become eczematous ; but they are aggravated by such forms of local irritation as tight garters. The rash is usually symmetrical, is first noticed on the limbs, but subsequently extends to the trunk, and in many cases attacks the tongue. It is occasionally accompanied by scaliness of the palms and soles. Itching is nearly always a constant symptom, and when present is very severe. The pruriginous condition resulting from the scratching often changes the character of the eruption. A tendency to constant relapses characterises this variety, and a history of previous attacks is often an important aid to diagnosis. Persons affected with this disease are generally about forty years of age, and are very rarely under twenty. As a rule there is little or no constitutional disturbance, but the general health may suffer as a result of repeated attacks.

LICHEN SCROFULOSORUM, LICHEN CIRCUMSCRIPTUS, LICHEN MARGINATUS.

Although Hebra describes under the name of L. scrofulosorum a variety of lichen which he believes to occur only in scrofulous subjects, there is reason to doubt whether the limitation thus indicated is altogether advisable; at all events, in this country we are accustomed to see cases which answer generally to his description, occurring also in others than scrofulous persons, and differing in certain characteristics to be mentioned hereafter.

In Hebra's variety all the papules appear about the same time in groups; they may vary greatly in colour, from that of the normal skin to a deep brownish-red. The shape of the groups is usually circular. The papules undergo no change, and are attended by but little local irritation. The eruption differs in its site from the other forms of lichen in being usually confined to the trunk and seldom attacking the limbs.

The English forms of Lichen scrofulosorum—viz. L. circumscriptus and L. marginatus—occur, as has already been pointed out, in persons who cannot be called scrofulous. The papules are grouped together in rings or patches, and a tendency to the former is very common. On the outer side of the rings the skin is normal, but within the circle is often slightly yellow, whilst the papules themselves are usually red. The eruption grows by extension of the rings, which as they increase in size meet other rings, and the papules disappearing at the point of contact, the so-called gyrate variety is produced. As the papules fade the skin is left stained with pigment. The usual site of this form of lichen is the back and chest. Some amount of itching is always present, which is aggravated by flannel vests.

Diagnosis.—The lichenous eruptions have to be distinguished from each other, from psoriasis, eczema, pityriasis rubra, tinea tonsurans, and pityriasis versicolor.

I

In the early stage it must be noticed that while lichen ruber begins with the development of red papules, which are scattered on any part of the body, but usually on the limbs, and are surmounted by small scales, the papules of lichen marginatus are of a lighter colour, are collected together in groups or rings, and appear more frequently on the trunk. Psoriasis begins with the formation of minute papules covered with white shining scales, situated mostly on the extensor surfaces of the limbs, and not aggregated together. Eczema begins with an eruption of small papules and vesicles, the latter containing clear fluid. The papules are never scaly, and are scattered irregularly, usually on the flexor surfaces of the limbs.

Later lichen ruber appears as red patches, consisting of aggregated papules, covered with thin scales. The patches never become moist. In lichen scrofulosorum and marginatus the papules appear in groups, that fade in the centre. In the more advanced stage of psoriasis large patches are formed by the coalescence of the original small spots through growth at their periphery ; they are all covered with white glistening, transparent scales, and in eczema the oozing from the surface gives rise to crusts, which are a most important diagnostic sign.

Pityriasis rubra at this stage can be diagnosed by the absence of infiltration, and by the fact that it extends uniformly over the greater part of the surface of the body. In the most advanced stage the eruption of lichen ruber consists of red patches covered with thin scales, the individual papules having disappeared. The skin is thickened, and the nails are affected. Lichen scrofulosorum never attacks the whole surface in the same manner as lichen ruber, and patches or rings rarely become scaly.

In the most advanced stage psoriasis can be distinguished from lichen ruber by the smaller amount of surface affected, and by the fact that healthy skin intervenes between the patches ; from lichen marginatus it can be easily diagnosed by the tendency of the rash in the latter to form rings with simply stained skin in the centre. Old-standing eczema can always be recognised by the crusts.

The eruption of pityriasis rubra can only be confounded with that of lichen ruber in the late stage, and can be distinguished from it by the absence of infiltration of the skin and severe constitutional symptoms of the former.

Lichen marginatus may be mistaken for ringworm of the body, but a microscopic examination of some of the epidermis will at once settle the doubt; the same disease may also bear some resemblance to pityriasis versicolor, but this can only occur when the rash is fading, and can be easily distinguished in the same way.

Prognosis.—There is comparatively little danger attending the lichenous diseases seen in this country, although some of them are very intractable, and last a long time on account of frequent relapses.

Morbid Anatomy. Lichen ruber.—On examining vertical sections of skin affected with lichen ruber, the epidermis is seen to be thickened and dried, especially on the hands and feet, but thin and scaly on other parts. The corium is also thickened and denser than normal, if the case is of old standing. The hyperæmia seen in life disappears after death. Under the microscope thin sections of the papules when first formed show merely enlargement of the root sheath at the base of the hair follicle, with numerous nodular outgrowths from it into the corium. Later the upper part of the root sheath may become enlarged, being, according to Hebra, pointed towards the hair follicle and expanded above, forming a series of concentric funnel-shaped envelopes round the hair. In the fully developed papules changes are found in other portions of the skin. The epidermis is thickened, and the rete Malpighii contains small round cells. The papillæ are enlarged, contain more round cells than normal, and have their fibrous tissue increased. The vessels in the papillary body and corium are enlarged and surrounded by small round cells. The root sheaths of the hair are thickened, as described above, and the arrectores pili are usually hypertro-

I 2

phied. The sebaceous and sweat glands do not seem to be primarily affected, but undergo degenerative changes as the disease progresses.

Lichen scrofulosorum.—On examining thin sections of the small papules at an early stage, the tissue round the vessels of the sebaceous and hair follicles affected is found to contain numerous leucocytes. This infiltration gradually extends upwards, and in the fully developed papules not only the follicular wall but the papillæ round the orifice of the hair follicle are filled with small round cells. In the later stages the exudation invades the hair follicle and sebaceous glands, and masses of cells are found between the root sheath and the follicular wall, in the substance of the root sheath itself, and in the rete Malpighii around the orifice of the follicle.

Treatment.—The treatment of lichen must be both local and constitutional. With regard to the former, the chief aim must be to allay the irritation, so as to afford rest, to remove all sources of irritation, such as flannel, and to apply soothing lotions and ointments composed of such drugs as hydrocyanic acid and weak preparations of tar. It is also necessary to pay great attention to cleanliness. In lichen scrofulosorum the local application of cod-liver oil is stated by Hebra to be of great value, but in applying this remedy care should be taken to keep it in constant contact with the skin. As regards internal remedies for lichen ruber or planus, there are no drugs so valuable as the various preparations of arsenic, but to produce any good result they must be taken in full doses and continued for a long period. It must be borne in mind that the use of this remedy must not be abandoned during the intervals of apparent cure, but must be continued with a view to prevent a relapse. If there is any proof of a scrofulous habit, cod-liver oil and iron must be given.

PRURIGO.

Definition.—Prurigo is a chronic papular disease of the skin, accompanied by intense irritation.

Symptoms.—The severe form of this disease described by Hebra as seen on the Continent is happily very rare in this country, only one or two cases having been reported.

The milder conditions known in England are prurigo mitis, occurring among children, and the relapsing prurigo of Hutchinson. Inasmuch as the prurigo of Hebra has many peculiarities in which it differs from the disease we understand by the same name, a short *résumé* of Hebra's description will therefore first be noticed.

Prurigo of Hebra.—The eruption first appears in the shape of sub-epidermic papules of the size of hemp seeds; they are but slightly elevated above the surface, of the same colour as normal skin, and are recognised more by the touch than the sight. They are always isolated, and may come out on all parts of the body, but, however severe, leave intervals of healthy skin. They are attended by intense itching, which causes the patient to scratch, giving rise to excoriations of the surface and the formation of small blood crusts on their summits. After this has lasted for some time the whole of the skin affected becomes hard, brawny, and darker in colour, owing to the deposit of pigment. As the disease progresses the normal furrows of the skin are seen to become deeper and farther apart; this is especially observable on the backs of the hands, the fingers, and the wrists. To the more severe form, which lasts the whole of life, the name of prurigo ferox is given. The parts most frequently attacked are the front and back of the chest, the whole of the back, loins, abdomen, and particularly the extensor surfaces of the limbs. The rash is less commonly present on the arms and thighs than on the forearms and legs, and on the whole more often attacks the lower than the upper extremities. Even in the most severe forms the flexor surfaces of the joints, the genitals, scalp, and face escape. Frequently eczema is produced as the result of the irritation, and in consequence the lymphatic glands become enlarged. Although the disease is never absolutely cured, at times the symptoms are so mitigated that it appears to have disappeared. Weather apparently has some effect on its intensity, for it is alway more severe in cold than in warm seasons. Prurigo is not congenital, but nearly always commences soon after birth.

Prurigo mitis.—Prurigo as we understand it is, as compared with the above disease, a simple malady. Although the objective symptoms in both varieties resemble each other, the English disease does not run such a protracted course as the German, and is in fact limited almost entirely to early life. The delicate skin of infants is usually in the first instance irritated by some local cause, such as flannel or the bites of parasites; as a result a papular eruption, together with some amount of urticaria, is developed, chiefly on the back and the extensor surfaces of the limbs. This is accompanied by severe itching, and when the child is old enough to scratch blood crusts are formed, which constitute an important characteristic of the disease. On passing the hand over the back the whole skin feels rough like a nutmeg grater.

Prurigo mitis usually occurs in delicate and badly nourished children, and is certainly more common among the poor, probably owing to their being more exposed to the causes above mentioned. The disease does not usually last longer than a few years, and is rarely seen in persons above the age of ten years.

Mr. Hutchinson has recently paid considerable attention to the prurigo of infants, and has made several important and interesting observations on its causation. He points out that there is considerable difference in the appearances of the ordinary eruption, which depends on the size of the papules and the amount of urticaria accompanying them, in some cases the papules being 'hard, rough, and dry like a nutmeg grater, while in other cases they are of larger size, like half-developed wheals of urticaria, with perhaps even some tendency to vesication,' and that there are besides two other distinct varieties to be distinguished. In one of these positive vesication takes place, and the palms and soles are affected. The history of the case leads to the belief that the child has in the first instance suffered from varicella. He states that it is not uncommon to find that the skin eruption commenced with a sudden outbreak of disease, which rapidly changed its character, and that, inasmuch as abortive varicella undoubtedly occurs, the first outbreak was probably due to this disease, which was not then recognised.

The ordinary prurigo eruption begins more gradually and varies in severity, being better in winter and worse in summer, and is due to the irritation produced by fleas or other parasites, which are more abundant in the warm than in the cold weather.

A pruriginous condition of skin may, however, also be induced by varicella or vaccination, which is not developed until the skin is subsequently irritated by flea-bites or some other local cause.

Prurigo may therefore be produced in one of three ways :—

1st. By the local irritation of fleas, or by wearing flannel, &c.

2nd. By these local causes acting on a skin which has been previously made susceptible to their influence by a previous attack of varicella or vaccination.

3rd. By the direct irritation of varicella itself without the intervention of any other exciting cause.

Relapsing Prurigo.—This disease, first described by Hutchinson, differs from the other forms of prurigo—first in the age at which it occurs, having a tendency to commence about puberty ; and secondly, in the colour of the papules, which are in this variety red. Together with the papular rash, which attacks most frequently the face, neck, and upper extremities, there is often an erythematous blush. Sometimes the rash leaves scars. Relapsing prurigo is attended with less itching than is the case in the other varieties, and does not produce the same hardness of skin as in Hebra's prurigo ; its distribution is the same as in the latter, inasmuch as it never attacks the palms, soles, genitals, or flexures of the joints.

Diagnosis.—Prurigo may under some circumstances be mistaken for scabies, phthiriasis, eczema, urticaria, pruritus, and erythema.

From scabies it may be distinguished by the different sites of the two diseases. The presence of the rash on the genitals and on the flexures of the joints will serve to eliminate prurigo. If a burrow can be discovered and the acarus produced, the diagnosis is of course easily settled; besides, pustules and constant itching are points in favour of scabies.

From pediculosis it may be diagnosed by the absence of pediculi.

From eczema it is often difficult to distinguish it, especially when the two diseases are combined. The character of the skin near the eruption assists the diagnosis, the reddening which accompanies eczema being entirely absent in prurigo. The scattered eruption, the blood crusts, and the tendency of the papules to bleed in prurigo are points of difference from eczema.

From urticaria and pruritus it can be recognised by the absence of papules in these two diseases.

From erythema (see Chapter IX., p. 102).

Prognosis.—The prognosis of Hebra's variety is unfavourable, and although the patient may live for years, his life is made utterly miserable by the intense itching. The prurigo of infants, due to a local cause, is curable when the cause is removed, but the duration of the disease is often protracted. The relapsing prurigo of Hutchinson is always a most obstinate form, lasting, in consequence of so many relapses, for years.

Morbid Anatomy.—On microscopic examination the changes found in Hebra's variety are described as follows :—

The epidermis is thickened considerably, especially in the rete Malpighii, where numerous small round cells are found. The papillary layer shows the papillæ enlarged, full of young cells, and their vascular loops dilated. Leucocytes are also found pretty freely scattered in the hair papilla and bulb, the root sheath, and in the corium around the follicle. In chronic cases spindle-shaped cells are found in the corium, and especially round the vessels.

Treatment.—Beyond attempting to alleviate the patient's

condition by attending to his general health and procuring sleep, nothing can be done to cure the variety described by Hebra. Since prurigo of children is often due to a local cause, this must be sought for and carefully removed; children, as a rule, outgrow prurigo, but considerable relief can be obtained from the use of tar baths, consisting of two or three or more teaspoonfuls of liquor carbonis detergens to a gallon of warm water. In such a bath the child should be kept for at least half an hour twice a day, and in the interval should be well anointed with a soothing ointment. For cachectic or strumous children cod-liver oil and steel wine should be prescribed. In the relapsing variety arsenic is of value.

CHAPTER XI.

Class I.—EXUDATIONES—*continued.*

3. *VESICULAR AND BULLOUS GROUP.*

Herpes febrilis, gestationis, iris—Hydroa—Pemphigus vulgaris, foliaceus.

HERPES.

Definition.—Herpes is an acute vesicular disease of the skin, which runs a rapid course and is accompanied by local irritation and sometimes by symptoms of constitutional disturbance.

Of the many varieties usually mentioned under this title only three are important enough to need special description— herpes febrilis, herpes gestationis, and herpes iris.

Symptoms.—*Herpes febrilis* may be described as a neurotic disease, and commonly occurs as a symptom of catarrh or of pneumonia, but may be due to any condition producing a rigor, such as the passing of a catheter. Whatever may be its cause, it always appears to be produced through the influence of the nervous system, and in all its forms the temperature is slightly increased, and the patient complains of headache and *malaise.* The eruption often precedes any constitutional symptom, and may occur on almost any part of the body, but its most common sites are the lips, tonsils, uvula, mucous membrane of the mouth, palate, and more rarely the face, ears, and tongue.

The eruption appears in groups, and lasts about seven or eight days. It consists of small papules, which become vesicular and which contain a clear fluid. After lasting two or three days this fluid becomes turbid, and is generally absorbed, though in some instances the vesicle bursts and crusts are formed. The vesicles themselves are situated on inflamed bases, and an itching or burning sensation always accompanies, and sometimes precedes by a few hours, the appearance of the eruption.

When herpes occurs on the lips, the vesicles are few in number, and rapidly coalesce and dry up into scabs; but when it appears on the mucous membrane of the mouth, they soon burst and leave a superficial ulceration. Again, when the vesicles form on the tonsils, uvula, or soft palate, they also burst, but leave white patches on the mucous membrane, which are liable to be mistaken for diphtheria, and this mistake is rendered more probable by a swelling of the tonsils which is occasionally seen at the same time. Although this disease usually occurs in isolated cases, a whole family is sometimes found to be attacked by it.

As a sub-variety of H. febrilis may be mentioned herpes progenitalis, in which the vesicles are developed on the prepuce, glands, or dorsum of the penis in the male, and on the labia or mons veneris in the female. These vesicles are generally few in number, and form scabs, which last but a short time and then drop off, leaving healthy skin; when, however, the vesicles are broken by scratching, small superficial ulcers result, which soon dry up and scab; and, further, it must be noticed that when there is much induration of the part it is difficult to distinguish the herpetic ulcer from the syphilitic chancre. Frequently also there is some amount of swelling, and the appearance of the eruption is often preceded by pain.

Herpes gestationis occurs in pregnant or parturient women, but is rarely seen in England. It has been recently described by Liveing and Bulkley. The rash is not purely vesicular, but consists of papules and vesicles of various sizes, from a pea to a bean, which appear in groups over the body, chiefly on the extremities. The eruption is preceded by and accompanied with severe itching, which continues after its disappearance, and by slight symptoms of constitutional disturbance and considerable pains in the limbs. Pigmentation is often left after the eruption disappears. This variety lasts some weeks, and is often prolonged by relapses.

Herpes iris, described by Willan as a separate variety, is characterised by the arrangement of the vesicles in rings round a single vesicle, and two or even three rings may be seen outside each other. They do not make their appearance simultaneously, but in successive circles, and those vesicles nearest the centre often subside during the growth of fresh vesicles at the periphery. It must not, however, be expected in herpes iris that all the vesicles are to be found arranged in this orbicular manner; it is sufficient to characterise the disease if some only are arranged in rings, whilst others appear in irregular crops, and it must be noticed also that, though they are usually discrete, they may coalesce and form bullæ. The disease itself lasts a variable time, usually from one to four weeks, according to the number of rings formed, and is not accompanied by any constitutional symptoms. Hebra points out the tendency of herpes and erythema to behave in a similar manner in producing multiform varieties, and that herpes circinatus results from herpes iris in the same way that erythema iris results from erythema annulare. The erythematous and herpetic rashes select the same sites, for they both occur most frequently on the backs of the hands and feet, at times on the limbs, in some instances as high as the arms or thighs, but hardly ever on the trunk. Hebra, indeed, goes so far as to say that, taking into consideration the similarity of the mode of development, the course and the seat of the two diseases, he is tempted to regard them as modifications of one and the same disease.

Diagnosis.—Herpes is not likely to be mistaken for any other disease, for the vesicles are larger than in eczema, and do not spread from the periphery, and are smaller than in pemphigus. The inflamed bases on which the vesicles are seated, the rapid course of the disease, and the sense of irritation which accompanies it, are sufficiently marked characteristics to prevent mistakes.

Prognosis.—The prognosis is always favourable, although the disease is occasionally protracted in the ringed variety.

Morbid Anatomy.—The morbid appearances are identical

with those found in pemphigus, and are therefore included in the description of the latter disease.

Treatment.—No local or constitutional treatment is known to affect the course of the disease.

HYDROA.

Definition.—In addition to these varieties of herpes, some mention must be made of a rare disease of a kindred nature, termed .hydroa by Bazin, who divides it into vesicular hydroa, vacciniform hydroa, and bullous hydroa. It is defined as a chronic disease of the skin, occurring in arthritic subjects, and characterised by groups of vesicles or bullæ.

Symptoms.—Vesicular hydroa first appears as small, round, deep red spots with well-defined edges, varying in size from a lentil to a threepenny piece, and sometimes surrounded by a rose-coloured area. The next day a vesicle forms in the centre of the spot, filled with a transparent yellow fluid, which in a day or two is absorbed from the centre, when the vesicle itself becomes a black scab.

Sometimes, especially during the cold weather, the fluid in the vesicle is so rapidly absorbed that there is only to be seen a white or yellow macula, formed by loose epidermis in the centre of a red disc. The eruption is usually accompanied by no symptoms of constitutional disturbance except feverishness. It generally makes its appearance on the backs of the hands, wrists, and front of the knees, but is occasionally found on the mouth, or even on the conjunctivæ. However, in the former case it does not occur on the mucous membrane till the third day, and then it is surrounded by a violet areola and scabs earlier.

Each outburst of vesicles lasts about four or five days, but, as they are constantly repeated, the disease usually continues for about three or four weeks, and even then relapses sometimes occur. Vesicular hydroa is a disease peculiar to gouty subjects of both sexes from twenty to thirty years of age, but generally attacks men. It is most common in spring and autumn, cold

and variations in temperature having a marked influence on its
appearance and course.

Vacciniform hydroa and bullous hydroa differ from the
vaiiety described in that the vesicles of the former disease
become umbilicated, and in the latter meet and form bullæ.

PEMPHIGUS.

Definition.—Pemphigus is characterised by the appearance
of bullæ in successive crops, terminating either in the absorption of the fluid or in bursting and giving rise to the formation
of ulcers.

Symptoms.—This disease differs according to the size, position, and behaviour of the bullæ and subsequent ulcers, but
may be divided into two chief varieties—pemphigus vulgaris
and pemphigus foliaceus, but the latter is rare.

Pemphigus vulgaris includes those forms which are most
frequently seen, and consists of two or three small bullæ situated
on slightly inflamed bases, which increase very rapidly until
they cover a surface of about two inches in diameter. They
are white, tense, and generally oval or round, but may lose
their shape by becoming confluent. The fluid in the bullæ is
at first clear and alkaline, but in a short time becomes turbid
and acid. A bulla may terminate by absorption of its fluid,
when nothing but the dried-up cuticle remains, or it may burst,
when it leaves an ulcerated surface, more or less covered with
crusts. A dark stain remains for some time to mark the site
of a bulla, and as the disease has a tendency to appear in successive crops, the skin gradually becomes more and more stained.
The bullæ may be scattered irregularly over the body, or may
be grouped together in circles or semicircles, from the circumference of which fresh bullæ grow at the same time as those in
the centre disappear. In other but rare cases red patches of
skin are found, in which the bullæ are badly defined or even
absent. All parts of the surface may be attacked with pemphigus, even the vagina and the rectum, but the head, palms,

and soles are almost always exempt. At the conclusion of the disease the skin becomes dry, and desquamation, often over a larger area than the actual site of the eruption, takes place. As a rule constitutional symptoms are not severe, depending solely on the amount of the eruption, but when the bullæ are of large size, and crops rapidly succeed each other, the itching becomes intolerable.

Pemphigus foliaceus differs from the preceding variety in colour, situation, and character of the blebs. The bullæ are of a red or yellow tint, and the vessels of the base can be seen through the fluid, which in this variety is small in quantity and does not distend the bulla. Around the first-formed bullæ others are developed, which eventually coalesce, while the fluid escapes and leaves crusts, the appearance of which is compared by Cazenave to that of flaky pie-crust. Although this condition is at first limited in area, it gradually spreads over the surface; and as there is no disposition for the part originally attacked to heal, a large portion of skin becomes affected, from which the smell is most offensive. The constitutional disturbance is slight at the commencement, but as the disease progresses feverishness, sleeplessness, and diarrhœa set in, and the patient finally succumbs.

Diagnosis.—Pemphigus is liable at all times to be mistaken for any disease in which vesicles or bullæ occur.

From erysipelas it may be distinguished by the extent of the inflamed surface and the defined margin of the former, while the latter has only a narrow areola around the vesicle, and by the fact that the constitutional symptoms which are characteristic of erysipelas do not occur in pemphigus.

From eczema simplex it may be distinguished by the smaller size of the vesicle in the former, and from scabies by absence of the burrows. Pemphigus foliaceus often presents great similarity to eczema rubrum, but the marked marasmus, pigmentation, and freedom from fibrous thickening of the skin in the former are the chief points of diagnosis between them.

Prognosis.—This is favourable if the eruption is limited to a small area, and if there be but few bullæ; but when they extend over a large surface, as in pemphigus foliaceus, death is the almost invariable result.

Morbid Anatomy.—Microscopic examination of the vesicles or bullæ shows the papillæ infiltrated with young cells, which extend also into the rete Malpighii in great numbers, and the capillaries are filled with blood. The sero-fibrinous exudation, escaping from the papillary layer, causes a separation of the epidermic layers; and as the fluid collects more abundantly opposite the apices of the papillæ, small columns of cells, elongated or variously altered in shape, give the vesicle a loculated appearance. A very abundant exudation, as in pemphigus, causes the cells to assume a spindled-shaped appearance, and finally the trabeculæ give way, leaving traces in the shape of delicate filaments attached to the roof and floor of the vesicle. The fluid in pemphigus consists at first of clear serum, in which numerous pale and only a few red corpuscles are found, but as the leucocytes soon undergo fatty degeneration, the contents assume an opalescent and then a more purulent appearance. Occasionally a large mixture of red corpuscles gives the serum a distinct sanguineous character.

Treatment.—This consists in improving the general condition, while local applications appear to exercise no influence on the course of the disease. A generous and nourishing diet is necessary, and for medicine arsenic in full and repeated doses is as important as quinine is in ague. Much relief also is afforded by frequent bathing, removing the crusts, and keeping the ulcers clean.

Little, however, can be done in pemphigus foliaceus but to combat the symptoms as they arise.

CHAPTER XII.

*Class I.—*EXUDATIONES—*continued.*

4. *ECZEMATOUS AND PUSTULAR GROUP.*

Eczema simplex—Acute : Eczema erythematosum, squamosum, papulatum, vesiculosum, pustulosum, fissum seu rimosum, rubrum,
Ecthyma—Chronic : Eczema capillitii, faciei, articulorum, manuum et pedum, crurale, genitale, corporis—Intertrigo—Porrigo
or Impetigo contagiosa.

ECZEMA—MOIST TETTER.

Definition.—Eczema is an acute inflammatory disease of the
skin, characterised by an erythematous papulo-vesicular or pustular eruption, which usually gives rise to a moist, reddened surface, and from which a serous discharge that stiffens linen exudes
freely. In the later stages it takes the form of a dull red or
brownish surface covered with scales. A sensation of burning
or marked itching accompanies it.

Symptoms.—The eruption may present various appearances,
as the disease, instead of going through the typical course above
indicated, may stop short at any one of the stages mentioned, or
may pass over or abbreviate some of them and then remain
stationary. In this way, instead of the red, excoriated, weeping
surface most commonly seen, a condition which is almost entirely erythematous, papular, vesicular, pustular, or squamous,
may be met with, and, according as one or other condition is
most prominent, several varieties have been described.

Various secondary changes may affect the portion of skin
suffering from eczema. Infiltration of the cutis and subcutaneous
tissue, cracks and fissures, abundant pus formation, superficial

K

ulceration, and the production of scabs are some of the phenomena most frequently met with. Scratching, in consequence of
the intense itching, often excites a renewed attack, and contri-
butes materially to the extension and persistence of the eruption.
Eczema may occur without any obvious cause in persons otherwise healthy; it may be excited by various local irritants, chemical, mechanical, thermal, &c.; it may affect those who are
gouty, syphilitic, or strumous, and in some instances it may be
hereditary.

Digestive, uterine, and nervous disorders may predispose to
or aggravate an attack of eczema, and should be taken into
account in the treatment.

According to its course and duration, eczema may be divided
into the *acute* and the *chronic* type, the latter being far the
most commonly met with; but local varieties, differing in appearance according to their site, require special description. Eczema
occurs in males more frequently than in females; of 6,798 cases
recorded by Hebra, McCall Anderson, and others 4,467 were
males, and only 2,331 females.

Acute Eczema is characterised by the occurrence of inflammatory redness and swelling of the skin, followed usually within
forty-eight hours by the eruption of numerous minute vesicles
containing clear yellowish serum, and accompanied with a
sensation of burning and tension. Within a week the vesicles
either dry up and desquamate or burst, leaving red oozing
points, or rapidly become pustular, giving rise, from desiccation,
to thin brownish or yellow crusts, which in separating leave a
reddish scaly surface, that itches slightly. A feeling of chilliness or slight pyrexia is usually the only constitutional symptom,
and within a fortnight the whole eruption may disappear. More
frequently, however, fresh crops are seen, either round the first or
on different parts of the body, attended by severe itching, which
causes violent scratching and produces excoriations. Successive acute attacks may thus prolong the disease, or it may pass
into a chronic form.

According to situation, the appearances vary somewhat.

On the face the redness and œdema of the skin are well marked, and may resemble erysipelas; the surface is, however, irregular and granulated, not uniformly smooth and shiny, as in the latter, and the disease is very prone to relapse and become chronic. On the hands and feet the eruption appears as a collection of small watery vesicle, with swelling and little or no redness at first, but they soon coalesce, and later on dry up; pain and tension are severe if the disease is extensive, but give place to itching as the eruption subsides. On the genitals swelling and redness form the main phenomena, the vesicles being usually small. Hebra states that in the male, while the penis remains dry and the vesicles rarely exceed a pin's point in size, on the scrotum they are larger, and on bursting give rise to an abundant discharge.

Repeated attacks usually cause the disease to become chronic.

Universal Acute Eczema is a rare variety, attended, according to Hebra, with but little constitutional disturbance besides a feeling of great chilliness. Different appearances are presented by the eruption, according to its site. On the face it produces the changes already described, on the trunk it resembles scarlatina which is beginning to desquamate, on the flexures of the limbs vesicles and raw weeping surfaces are more common, while on the scalp the abundant scabs which are produced by the secretion from the vesicles, and retained by the hair, form a foul-smelling, offensive-looking mass.

Chronic Eczema presents appearances of the same nature as those met with in the acute disease—viz. papules, vesicles, pustules, crusts, and extensive red moist and weeping or dry scaly surfaces.

The frequent relapses and the persistence of the disease cause a more abundant serous discharge, and the prolonged infiltration of the skin often gives rise to hypertrophy of the papillary body, with sclerosis of the cutis and subdermic tissues.

According as one or other lesion predominates, we may have *eczema erythematosum*, with simple inflammatory redness of the skin, followed by desquamation; *eczema squamosum* (often de-

K 2

scribed as pityriasis rubra), with abundant formation of scabs
on a reddened, infiltrated basis, with little or no discharge ;
eczema papulosum (frequently termed lichen eczematodes, &c.),
with an eruption of small red aggregated papules ; *eczema vesiculosum*, the vesicles being either small and rapidly bursting, or
larger and by confluence forming bullæ where the skin is thick
and dense, as on the hands and feet ; *eczema pustulosum*, where,
either from the beginning or soon after their appearance, the
vesicles become pustular, and, drying up, give rise to brownish,
yellowish, or black crusts, conditions which have been raised to
the rank of a new and separate disease under the name of
impetigo contagiosa ; *eczema fissum seu rimosum*, where
numerous cracks of varying depth in an erythematous dry or
moist surface occur in places where the skin is normally thrown
into folds ; and *eczema rubrum*, where the red, infiltrated, excoriated surface, usually discharging profusely, is well developed.
This last form is accompanied by severe burning heat, and later
on by intense itching ; constitutional symptoms—fever, headache,
and digestive derangement—are well marked, and the surface
pre ents numerous bright red points of hyperæmia, from which
fluid keeps continually exuding, like the drops of water on the
surface of salt butter (Hutchinson). The disease described as
ecthyma consists of an eruption of large flattened pustules on a
red, indurated, slightly raised base, giving rise frequently to dark
brown, dense crusts and unhealthy, sloughy ulcers ; it is merely
a form of pustular eczema occurring in debilitated cachectic persons living under bad hygienic conditions.

Of the local varieties of chronic eczema the following will
now be described :—

1. Eczema capillitii.
2. Eczema faciei.
3. Eczema articulorum.
4. Eczema manuum et pedum.
5. Eczema crurale.
6. Eczema genitale.
7. Eczema corporis.

1. *Eczema capillitii.*—In eczema of the scalp, owing to the presence of the hair, which becomes glued together by the sero-purulent discharge, a dense matted crust may be produced if the disease is left to run its course unchecked, until the entire scalp is affected. Pus, mingled with sebaceous secretion from the numerous glands, forms beneath the crusts, and pediculi, their ova, and even maggots may find a resting-place in the filthy, stinking mass. When occurring in discrete spots and in clean people the discharge and crusts are constantly removed, and the disease is easily recognised.

In the later stages, when the crusts have separated and the discharge is less in quantity, a red, infiltrated surface covered with numerous scales adherent to the hairs is seen.

This variety is usually pustular, occurs most often in children, and may persist for years if neglected. Subcutaneous abscesses and glandular enlargements are not unfrequently met with, especially in strumous children. In chronic cases there is some loss of hair, speedily renewed, however, when the disease is cured, except in neglected cases where profuse suppuration under the scabs has destroyed the hair follicles.

2. *Eczema faciei.*—Eczema of the face, when it affects the hairy parts, resembles the former variety in the liability to the production of shallow pustules with a hair passing through them, which dry up and form yellow, greenish, or brown crusts. On removal they leave a red moist or scaly surface. In chronic cases the hair follicles become more deeply involved, as in sycosis; the skin is dusky red, and thickened and permanent alopecia is apt to follow, from the destruction of the hair bulbs. Pain and burning heat, with later on some itching, accompany the eruption.

Eczema of the eyelashes, or tinea tarsi, frequently confounded with inflammation of the Meibomian glands, is merely a local eczema implicating the hair follicles and glands, and is always accompanied by itching. Redness, swelling, and excoriations, and scabbing of the margins of the lids, with partial or complete loss of the eyelashes, may be produced by it.

Eczema of the nostrils usually terminates in the formation of a thick scab, which felts together the margins and blocks up the orifice. The continual pus formation under it causes often an erysipelatous swelling of the mucous membrane or skin of the nose.

On the smooth parts of the face eczema is usually symmetrical, unless produced by purely local causes.

Eczema of the ears may occur merely as a moist fissure at the reflection of the auricle from the mastoid process, or as a weeping or crusted red surface at the back of the auricle, on the lobule, or elsewhere. The skin is prone to excessive swelling and discharge, which either drips away constantly or dries up, forming stalactiform crusts. Hearing, always somewhat impaired, is made much worse when the meatus is affected and blocked up more or less completely by crusts and ceruminous discharge.

Eczema of the lips may present either a red, scaly, infiltrated or a moist surface. There is often marked œdema, with painful fissures or large yellow crusts.

On the cheeks and forehead large yellow crusts, looking like dried honey—which gained for the disease in this site the names of crusta lactea and melitagra flavescens—are most commonly seen.

3. *Eczema articulorum* occurs on the flexor surfaces of the limbs, and leads to slight contraction, with great pain on moving the subjacent joint. The skin, red, much infiltrated, and oozing or crusted, is traversed by numerous fissures, following the lines of the normal folds of skin, causing the application of the name eczema fendillé. Eczema rubrum occurs most frequently in these situations.

4. *Eczema manuum et pedum.*—The fissured variety of eczema is here most common, especially on the palms and soles, where the skin presents a dry, inelastic, thickened appearance, itches considerably, and is traversed by numerous deep, painful fissures. The vesicular form, with large blebs, pustules, crusts, or moist surfaces, may also occur. Local irritants—

water, sugar, lime, soda, soap, dyes, &c.—are the most common causes of eczema restricted to the hands or feet; hence the so-called 'grocer's itch,' 'baker's itch,' &c., are merely local varieties of eczema.

5. *Eczema crurale* is often modified, and its typical features concealed, by conditions peculiar to its site, such as varicose veins, ulcers, scars, pigment patches, and œdema, leading to chronic dermatitis.

The disease hence arises sometimes around a varicose ulcer or scar, sometimes on a pigmented patch, and at others the œdema appears as if secondary to the skin affection; but in all cases eczema, whether as simplex, rubrum, or squamosum, is easily recognised.

6. *Eczema genitale*, occurring in the chronic form, affects in the male the scrotum and penis either together or separately. On the penis it appears as raised red transverse lines; on the dorsum it is most marked when the skin is stretched, with a moister red area on the under surface of the organ. Though itching is severe, and induces much scratching and excoriation, there is but little discharge. On the scrotum it may occur as an abraded red surface, comparatively free from infiltration, or as an irregular fissured or greatly hypertrophied elephantoid mass in inveterate cases, exuding an abundant sticky discharge, which, as it decomposes and dries up, becomes extremely offensive.

On the female genitals the disease affects the labia majora chiefly, and may extend to the nymphæ and vulva or to the adjacent parts of the thigh and abdomen, and takes usually the form of eczema rubrum. When affecting the mucous membrane it causes an abundant blennorrhagic discharge, resembling that of gonorrhœa, and there is usually much burning and itching. Appearing about the anus, it leads to the formation of painful itching fissures in the direction of the normal radiating folds of skin. There is often slight prolapsus ani, and the discharge is abundant and offensive.

7. *Eczema corporis*, presenting the general characters of the

disease as described on p. 130, has some special peculiarities
when it attacks the navel and nipples. The nipple and the
adjacent areola are denuded of epidermis, red, swollen, moist,
and painful; and crusts may form, under which either healing
goes on or increased secretion, which oozes under or through
the scab, and is accompanied by severe itching and pain. It may
spread gradually to the surrounding skin, and is very obstinate ;
but, once cured, it leaves but little permanent damage behind.

On the umbilicus it takes either the ordinary form of
eczema rubrum or impetiginosum, or that of an œdematous projecting red surface denuded of epidermis, and discharging freely
or covered with a yellowish or greenish brown scab.

Eczema intertrigo occurs in the axillæ, between the nates,
between the mammæ and chest, and in other places where folds
of skin secrete much moisture and rub together, and appears as
a moist, red, and tender surface, sometimes slightly excoriated.

The so-called *Eczema marginatum,* formerly held to be a
special variety of eczema, has now been shown to be merely one
of the manifestations of ringworm of the body.

Diagnosis.—Eczema in one or other of its forms may sometimes be mistaken for the following diseases :—erythema, erysipelas, lichen ruber, herpes febrilis, miliaria, scabies, pemphigus
foliaceus, psoriasis, pityriasis rubra.

In *Erythema* the smooth isolated spots which generally
appear on the backs of the hands, the sharply-defined edges, the
absence usually of vesicles, discharge, and crusts, and the slight-
ness of subjective symptoms, form a ready means of separation
from eczema erythematosum or papulatum, which have a rough
—often vesiculate—surface shading off into the surrounding
skin.

Erysipelas is separated from acute eczema by the marked
pyrexia, which begins usually with rigors, by the smooth surface with well-defined edge, and the rapid spreading of the
patches, by the affection of the lymphatics, and the greater
severity of the burning heat and pain. Erysipelas may, however, supervene on an attack of eczema.

Lichen ruber, which in aggregated patches may resemble eczema papulatum or squamosum, never becomes at any stage vesicular, and the isolated, flat-topped, shiny, solid papules that are found round the margin of the patch are quite characteristic.

Herpes febrilis, which occurs most commonly on the lips and prepuce, is distinguished from eczema of the same parts by the larger size and longer duration of the vesicles, and the absence of infiltration and itching. The vesicles dry up in a few days, and are not succeeded by fresh crops, as in eczema.

Miliaria differs from eczema in the fact that the vesicles occur in groups, usually on the abdomen and thorax, in the course of some febrile disorder. The eruption is of short duration, and is unattended by itching. In eczema, on the other hand, there is little or no constitutional disturbance, the vesicles are aggregated on a red base, there is marked itching, and the disease tends to become chronic.

In *Scabies* the vesicles, pustules, and scabs which are produced by the irritation of the parasite, or the itching and scratching that it excites, are undistinguishable from those of eczema. Careful examination will usually show near the pustules the little dark lines of the burrows, with a terminal dilatation from which the acarus can often be extracted. The appearance of the disease on the hands and feet, wrists and abdomen, is also a suspicious circumstance.

Pemphigus foliaceus presents an appearance that is often difficult to distinguish from general eczema which discharges only slightly and is becoming scaly. The peculiar cachexia, the diarrhœa and marked weakness, and the pigmentation of the skin, together with the tendency of pemphigus foliaceus to begin on the front of the trunk, contrast markedly with the absence of cachexia and pigmentation, the itching and the tendency to infiltration and sclerosis of the skin, in eczema.

The condition known as eczema squamosum may sometimes be mistaken for *Psoriasis*. The latter affects mainly the extensor surfaces instead of the flexors, as in eczema. The scales, thick, adherent, and silvery, are seated on abruptly-defined, dark red patches, while in eczema the scales are thin, loose, not silvery, and the bright red patches merge more gradually into the adjacent skin. Psoriasis is dry throughout, while chronic eczema always discharges at one period of its existence.

Pityriasis rubra, regarded by some as merely a variety of eczema, differs, according to McCall Anderson, in the uniform redness and defined margin of the eruption, extending gradually to cover the whole surface, in the rapid exfoliation of large scales, in the burning heat and comparatively slight itching, and in the absence of any considerable infiltration, while the punctate appearance of the skin, the papules, vesicles, and crusts are quite wanting.

Eczema of the hands and feet may, by the confluence of several vesicles under the thick palmar cuticle, acquire bullæ, which resemble those of *Pemphigus.* Small vesicles and a definite eczematous eruption are usually present in the neighbourhood, and prevent the possibility of error.

Both *Psoriasis* and a *tertiary squamous syphilide* affecting the palms and soles may be indistinguishable from eczema, and only the discovery of evidences of these diseases on other parts of the body can determine the diagnosis.

The diagnosis of the principal diseases of the scalp is given in the following table.

DIFFERENTIAL DIAGNOSIS BETWEEN ECZEMA CAPITIS AND SEBORRHŒA, PSORIASIS, VESICO-PUSTULAR SYPHILIDE, TINEA TONSURANS, AND FAVUS OF THE SCALP.

ECZEMA	SEBORRHŒA	PSORIASIS	VESICO-PUSTULAR SYPHILIDE	TINEA TONSURANS	FAVUS
1. Most frequent in children, in the debilitated or strumous.	1. Usually in adults.	1. Most often in healthy persons, rarely in strumous.	1. Usually in adults only.	1. Frequent in children.	1. No special proneness in strumous.
2. Often attacks the whole scalp. Ulcers if any, superficial; crusts thick, yellowish, brittle; pus, epithelium, and granular matter. Seated on red, infiltrated, moist, often excoriated surface, which shades off gradually into healthy skin and itches excessively.	2. Crusts are thin, oily, can be kneaded into masses; consist chiefly of sebum and epithelium on a smooth, oily surface; no, or only slightly, red, and non-excoriated or infiltrated; itching only slight.	2. Eruption usually white, scaly, and silvery; dry from onset and throughout course; red base, only slightly infiltrated, and itching only slight.	2. In small patches usually; often deep ulcers with sloughy bases.	2. Patches usually circular, deficient in hair; crusts, &c., not necessarily present; itching slight.	2. Round, dry, sulphur yellow, cup-shaped crusts, penetrated by dull brittle hairs, with abrupt edges and often bald patches.
3. Syphilitic history and phenomena only accidental, if present at all.	3. Usually no specific phenomena.	3. Usually no specific history.	3. Usually a history of primary syphilis, and presence of alopecia, nocturnal pains, &c.		
4. Distinct eczema often on other parts of body, on flexor surfaces or behind the ears.	4. Usually only slight, oily crusting on face near scalp.	4. Well-marked scaly patches usually present on extensor surfaces of elbows and knees.	4. Syphilitides, squamous, pustular, tubercular, &c., with coppery colour, usually present on body.	4. Ringworm of body (tinea circinata) often present.	4. Cupped yellow crusts may be found on hairy parts of the body.
5. Hair healthy, occasionally falling out; no parasite.	5. Hairs often drop out.	5. Hairs only slightly affected.	5. Hairs fall out freely, and incurable alopecia may result.	5. Hairs twisted, thickened, whitish, broken off short, easily extracted; filled with trichophyton tonsurans.	5. Hairs dull, dry, brittle, easily extracted, loaded with achorion Schönleinii.
6. Non-contagious.	6. Non-contagious.	6. Non-contagious.	6. Communicable by inoculation, which produces a hard chancre, followed by constitutional symptoms.	6. Contagious.	6. Contagious.

Prognosis.—In itself the disease alone is never fatal. An ordinary attack of acute eczema runs through its various stages and subsides, leaving little or no trace within a week or ten days. Fresh crops of eruption arising near the original patch, or on distant parts of the body, may appear in succession, and prolong the disease for many weeks, verging gradually into the chronic form. The latter, with alternations, retrogressions, and relapses, may persist for months or even years.

Among the local varieties of chronic eczema the more limited the area of the patch, the more obstinately does it persist in spite of treatment.

Morbid Anatomy.—Microscopic examination shows that the papular and vesicular stages are produced as follows :—Abundant transudation of plasma and cells gives rise to an enlargement and elongation of the papillæ, which contain numerous leucocytes. Biesiadecki describes a numerous plexus of spindle-shaped cells between the ordinary rete elements which they enclose in their meshes. The cells of the stratum lucidum next enlarge and burst, and fluid collecting between the rete and horny layers produces a vesicle containing serum and leucocytes. The vascular plexuses of the papillary layer, and of the hair and gland follicles, are hyperæmic. In chronic cases there is more or less cell infiltration of the cutis, most dense around the vessels, which gradually extends down into the subcutaneous tissues, and, by the production of spindle cells and new-formed fibrous tissue around the fat cells and capillaries, causes a sclerosis of the skin resembling that met with in elephantiasis. The columnar rete cells contain brown pigment, and in the corium thin strands of pigment mark the sites of obliterated vessels.

Treatment.—In the constitutional treatment the main indications are—first, to remove or modify any condition which predisposes to the occurrence of the disease ; and, secondly, to give sufficient nutritious, easily digested food, and to forbid the use of stimulants.

Hence the action of the bowels must be regulated by occa-

s:onal doses of the aperient mineral waters, such as Carlsbad or
Hunyadi Janos. Gouty symptoms must be combated by col-
chicum and alkalies, and for strumous children cod-liver oil and
iron is required.

In the acute forms antimony is of the greatest value, and,
according to Dr. Cheadle, often does good when all other reme-
dies fail. It should be given in doses of $\frac{1}{12}$ to $\frac{1}{6}$ of a grain two
or three times a day. In the chronic forms arsenic, iron,
quinine, and strychnine are of use as tonics, but none of them
have any specific action on the disease.

In local treatment the indications are—

1. To use sedatives only, or mild unirritating applications
during the acute stages, or in acute exacerbations of the chronic
form.

2. To remove thoroughly all scales or scabs before applying
local remedies.

In the stage of heat and tension dressing with simple cold
soft water, or with a lead and opium lotion, is the best remedy
to apply, but soap of all kinds should be avoided. Dusting-
powders of starch, oxide of zinc, or chalk may be tried. Crusts
should be removed by softening them with oil or a bread and
water poultice, and then scraping them off gently. After clean-
ing the part with oatmeal paste, or with simple water, the surface is ready for local applications. The best are *mild* solutions
of tar or weak preparations of mercury ; of the former the most
convenient form is Wright's liquor carbonis detergens. It is
an alcoholic solution of coal tar, and mixes well with water ;
3ij to the eight ounces of water is the strength which should
be used at first, and should be gradually increased if the lotion
is borne without pain or smarting. The following prescription
from the Pharmacopœia of the Skin Hospital, Blackfriars, is of
considerable value in allaying the itching and preventing the
formation of fresh scabs :—

℞ Acetate of lead	.	.	.	.	.	grains 10
Oxide of zinc	.	.	.	.	.	„ 20
Calomel	.	.	.	.	.	„ 10
Citrine ointment	.	.	.	.	.	„ 20
Palm oil	.	.	.	.	.	℥ss
Benzoated lard to	.	.	.	.	℥j

In the chronic, inveterate, and localised varieties blister-ing in successive small portions may be tried, or the vigorous application of Hebra's spiritus saponatus alkalinus. Tar, or various forms of it and substances got from it, are most useful in the scaly forms of eczema; but if used at all in the acute stages it should be with great caution, as they are apt to pro-duce fresh outbreaks of the disease. The substance itself, oil of cade, ol. rusci, or ol. fagi, may either be applied pure, or in ointments containing 1 to 8 or 12 parts.

In *Eczema capitis*, after removing scabs by oil, poultices, and washing, the following ointment may be applied with advantage :—

Bisulphuret of mercury	.	.	.	.	grains 6
Red precipitate .	.	.	.	.	.	„ 6
Creosote	.	.	.	.	.	.	m 2
Lard or vaseline	.	.	.	.	.	℥j

(Skin Hospital.)

Eczema faciei.—After cutting short the hair and removing the scabs, an ointment of oleate of bismuth or zinc, one part to two of vaseline, should be applied on lint, and retained in posi-tion by a flannel mask.

Eczema in the ears should be treated by removal of the crusts, and by brushing out the meatus cautiously with a potash solution—5 to 10 grains to the ounce.

Eczema of the eyelids, or tinea tarsi, should be treated by removal of the crusts, epilation, and the application of one of the mild mercurial ointments before mentioned.

In *Eczema manuum et pedum* wrap the affected part with strips of lint covered with zinc ointment, and apply some tar or other stimulant when the fissures are healed. Vulcanised indiarubber gloves, as recommended by Dr. McCall Anderson, are of considerable value when the cuticle is very thick and hard.

In *Eczema of the legs*, after removing the crusts and dressing the ulcers with a weak tar or lead and opium lotion, strap the limbs with stout plaster, or better still with Martin's elastic bandage.

In *Eczema of the genitals* bathing with water, and dressing with a glycerine lotion, such as—

> Glycerine . . . . ♏24
> Oil of bitter almonds . . . . . ♏½
> Water to . . . . ℥j
> Diluted with 1 to 3 parts of water (*Skin Hospital*)—

in the day, and well smearing the part just before bed time with the following ointment, will tend to remove the disease :—

> Acetate of lead . . . . . grains 10
> Liq. carbonis detergens . . . ♏10 or 15
> Vaseline . . . . ℥j

Eczema intertrigo requires little treatment beyond washing with soft water and the use of some dusting powder or vaseline, together with the careful separation of the parts by means of soft lint.

In *Eczema of the nipple* painting with tincture of catechu is useful after the removal of the crusts, and in very obstinate cases Hebra recommends the thorough application of a strong potash solution as a last resource.

PORRIGO—IMPETIGO CONTAGIOSA.

Definition.—A local disease of the skin, communicable by inoculation, excited most commonly by accidental irritation, and characterised by an eruption of flat vesicles, which rapidly change into pustules and dry into yellow friable crusts.

Symptoms.—From scratching or from any accidental irritation of the skin there arises, usually on the face or head, but sometimes on the hands, an eruption of isolated small vesicles, which soon become pustular and then dry into yellow scabs. These scabs vary in size from a split pea to a shilling, and appear as if 'stuck on,' since there is no inflammatory areola round them. Dr. Tilbury Fox, who first distinguished the disease as a separate affection, states that the eruption is generally preceded by a slight pyrexia, and by *malaise* and sensations of chilliness; also that it is accompanied by severe itching, which is particularly troublesome at night.

On removing the scabs a reddened base secreting a gummy, purulent fluid, which does not stiffen linen like that of eczema, is seen, and as the disease abates the scabs fall off from the erythematous base and the red spots gradually fade.

When the head is affected the posterior cervical glands are apt to enlarge, and if the disease be neglected pediculi may be present among the scabs. The disease is spread from one part of the body to another, and from one person to another, by the direct inoculation of the pus.

Diagnosis.—The eruption of discrete vesicles, which soon become pustules and scabs, the absence of serous discharge and the presence of pus, the inoculability, the contagiousness and the slight pyrexia which precedes it, are the points which are supposed to separate porrigo from eczema.

Prognosis.—The disease runs an acute course, and usually lasts about a fortnight. It may be prolonged by successive eruptions, but is never dangerous to life.

Morbid Anatomy.—The conditions met with resemble those of eczema. Fungus elements have been found in the crusts, but not in the contents of the vesicles, so that they are probably accidental.

Treatment.—The removal of the scabs by oiling and poultices, and the subsequent application of a mild mercurial ointment, or a carbolic acid lotion (1 in 20), to destroy the infective character of the pus, are the remedies that are needed to effect a cure.

CHAPTER XIII.

Class I.—EXUDATIONES—*continued.*

5. *SQUAMOUS GROUP.*

Pityriasis rubra—Psoriasis vulgaris—Pityriasis.

PITYRIASIS RUBRA.

Definition.—Pityriasis rubra is a chronic scaly disease, characterised by an intense reddening of the skin, which soon extends over the whole body, but which is not accompanied by any infiltration or thickening.

Symptoms.—Pityriasis rubra is a somewhat rare disease. Its chief characteristic is an intense reddening of the skin, which gradually extends over the whole surface, but fades on pressure. There is no infiltration or thickening of the reddened area, but the affected part is covered with loose scales of epidermis, which are shed in enormous quantities, often in large flakes, and the nails become opaque and irregular.

The reddening is much increased by heat, while cold, on the other hand, gives it a blue tint. At a late stage of the disease the colour becomes lighter and of a yellow or brown hue, which fades after death, when the skin resumes its normal appearance. At no time is the itching at all severe, and constitutional symptoms are for a long time absent; but in the later stages of the disease the skin becomes extremely tender, the appetite becomes impaired and the body emaciated, until death results.

The above description applies to the disease first separated from other affections by Hebra. It is right to mention, however, that several modern observers are of the opinion that it is

L

merely an abnormal form of eczema, in which there is little or no exudation. Hutchinson believes that the essential features of the disease are 'its occurrence in healthy persons, its proneness to become universal, and its non-amenability to treatment.' 'If, then, a person in good health should, without obvious cause, become the subject of a skin disease which should spread rapidly and very widely, involving the whole surface, and this eruption should prove to be uninfluenced by treatment, I would not care much whether the skin was dry or moist, whether it began as vesicles, papules, or erythematous patches, whether it were pruriginous or not. Such a malady would be probably, so far as causes are concerned, a close ally of pityriasis rubra' ('Clinical Lectures,' 1879). The hard and fast lines drawn by Hebra, which would exclude from the category of pityriasis rubra all cases which do not conform exactly to the above description, cannot be sustained in practice, because cases differing somewhat from the typical form of pityriasis rubra, both in the character and the severity of the eruption and in the nature of their course, are not unfrequently met with.

Diagnosis.—From psoriasis and lichen ruber it may be at once separated by the absence of any infiltration, while the intense reddening of the surface enables it to be distinguished from pityriasis simplex or ichthyosis. The absence of moisture marks a difference from all varieties of eczema, and, further, the large extent of surface involved, the tenderness of the skin, and the absence of the characteristic papules definitely separate it from eczema squamosum, which is, moreover, essentially a local affection, while pityriasis rapidly becomes general.

Lupus erythematosus is said by Hebra to resemble pityriasis rubra both in the reddening of the skin and the production of epithelial scales, but the former is limited to the face, and is attended with ' enlargement of the mouths of the hair sacs and sebaceous glands, which are also plugged with masses of hardened sebum.'

Prognosis.—The prognosis in this disease is very unfavourable, and the majority of cases terminate fatally.

Morbid Anatomy.—In early stages the microscopic examination shows little besides scaling of the horny layer, with moderate serous and cellular infiltration of the rete and of the papillary layer. In other cases there is marked atrophy of the whole skin, the rete and the papillary layer are atrophied, the horny layer thin and scaly, the connective-tissue fibres of the corium thickened, and elastic fibres more numerous. There is also considerable deposit of pigment, and the hair follicles, sweat and sebaceous glands, are much wasted.

Treatment.—No treatment has been found of any material use in checking the course of this disease, but the employment of tepid baths and the application of oil and emollient ointments is recommended by Hebra.

PSORIASIS VULGARIS.

Definition.—Psoriasis is a chronic disease of the skin, characterised by the production of white silvery scales on hyperæmic bases.

Symptoms.—The eruption begins with congestion of the papillæ of the skin, giving rise to an increased production of epidermic cells in the form of a quantity of minute elevations, which increase in size and are separated from each other by healthy skin. When these are of the size of pins' heads, the name *psoriasis punctata* is given to the eruption; as they develope they have the appearance of drops of mortar, and it is then known as *psoriasis guttata*; a further increase by growth of the periphery brings them to the size of coins, when the rash is described as *psoriasis nummularis*. While the patches first formed in this way develope in size, others are continually beginning, until patches of all sizes are to be seen. These patches of diseased skin have a tendency to heal in their centres, while extension takes place at their margins, and as a result rings are formed, the circumferences of which vary in thickness according to the size of the patches, since the healing process in the centre takes place more rapidly than the growth at the margins. To this variety the name of *psoriasis circinata* or *lepra* is usually given. Frequently two rings come in contact with each other at the edges, thus forming the figure 8; or three rings will meet, producing a trefoil. Often, however, the circles are not complete, and as a result a quantity of wavy lines are formed. This variety is known as *psoriasis gyrata* or *figurata*. The rings never overlap each other, each presenting an impenetrable barrier to the extension of contiguous rings. The name of *psoriasis universalis* is given to the eruption when the patches increase in size, coalesce, and cover the whole of the body. This is very rarely met with, and even when it does occur a considerable portion of healthy skin remains unattacked and intervenes between the diseased patches. When the thickening of the skin and the growth of epidermic cells is very marked, the eruption is called *psoriasis inveterata*. A further form has been described by McCall Anderson under the name of *psoriasis rupioides*, owing to the special prominence of the patches, which are usually larger than in psoriasis guttata. 'The accumulation of the epidermis takes place to an unusual extent, so that on many of the patches it assumes the shape of large conical crusts marked by concentric rings.' When the crusts are removed no ulceration remains, but 'a slightly elevated dusky red surface is exposed to view, which sometimes bleeds a very little.'

Although when psoriasis first appears there is little discoloration of the skin, it soon becomes raised and of a marked red colour, which as time goes on grows darker. At a later stage the scales are shed, leaving the red patches still raised but bare. At a further period, when the disease commences to heal, the patch becomes less and less elevated, and the colour lighter and lighter, till eventually the eruption fades, leaving the skin perfectly normal and not stained with pigment.

Psoriasis, as a rule, is attended by some amount of local irritation, and the scratching which results leads to the formation of small blood crusts. Hebra has pointed out that these will always be found on the edge of the patch as well as in its centre, and states that the older patches only itch at their margins, and concludes therefore that the itching only occurs while the eruption is growing.

Psoriasis may occur on any part of the body, but the tips of the elbows, the fronts of the knees, and the head are specially liable to be affected. It may be limited to the knees and elbows without attacking other parts, but if the rest of the body is implicated these regions are but rarely exempt. When the head is attacked, the eruption extends beyond the part covered with hair and forms a ring round the forehead and ears. Often the disease penetrates into the meatus of the ear, and thus produces deafness. Psoriasis is never seen on the mucous membranes or the red margins of the lips, and but rarely on the palms and soles. The nails are sometimes subjected to the action of the disease, and then become thick, friable, and of a brown colour.

Psoriasis of the scalp produces no changes either in the colour or structure of the hair, although it causes it to be shed more freely than is naturally the case.

Although much difference of opinion exists regarding the conditions that lead to the production of psoriasis, there is no reason for believing that climate, habits of life, special occupations, exposure to cold, uncleanliness, diathesis, temperament, pregnancy, mental emotion, syphilis, gout or other diseases, or even sex, race, or age, have any influence on its origin. It is undoubtedly hereditary, and it is comparatively rare to find psoriasis in one member of a family without finding it in another.

Diagnosis. — Psoriasis may be confounded with seven diseases—

1. Squamous syphilide (see Chap. VIII., p. 90).
2. Lichen ruber (see Chap. X., p. 114).
3. Eczema squamosum (see Chap. XII., p. 137).
4. Pityriasis rubra (see p. 146).
5. Pityriasis can be distinguished from psoriasis by the con-

trast of the thick white scales of the latter with the thin dark scales of the former, and by the absence of thickening of the skin in pityriasis.

6. Ichthyosis is easily recognised by the absence of the redness of the skin and the white silverlike scales peculiar to psoriasis, and by the fact of the disease affecting the whole surface and being congenital.

7. Tinea circinata occasionally bears a rough resemblance to psoriasis, but it does not attack the knees and elbows, its scales are not silvery, and microscopic examination will enable the parasite to be distinguished.

Prognosis.—Psoriasis is not a fatal disease, but is exceedingly obstinate, though to some extent amenable to treatment, and it is liable to relapse.

Morbid Anatomy.—Thin sections from a patch which has not lasted long show the epidermis much thickened, especially the rete, which is soft and contains many leucocytes. The papillæ also are infiltrated with numerous leucocytes, which fill up the connective-tissue meshwork, and the vessels are dilated, while their adventitia is thickened and loaded with cells.

Old patches often show thickening and induration of the whole corium, with vascular dilatation, serous and cellular infiltration, and some deposit of pigment in the branched cells as deep as the subcutaneous fatty tissue.

In psoriasis inveterata the papillæ on the back of the sacrum, and over the olecranon and the upper part the tibia, become enlarged and sclerosed, forming hard warty masses as in ichthyosis. The scales are made up of masses of cells from the stratum lucidum, which, as in other conditions producing inflammatory overgrowth, have not undergone the usual horny transformation, but have simply dried up and become pervaded with air. To this their friable consistency and their silvery colour, as well as the readiness with which they separate from the hyperæmic papillary layer, are due.

Treatment.—The treatment of psoriasis consists in the use of constitutional and local remedies. Of the constitutional remedies no drug has proved of such service as arsenic, which should be given in increasing doses until the eruption begins to disappear, and then continued in small quantities for a great length of time.

The alkaline treatment has been said to be attended with success, but it is of doubtful value. It is given in the form of liquor potassæ, in doses of twenty or thirty drops three times daily. McCall Anderson has seen much benefit derived from the use of carbonate of ammonia, which should be given in doses increasing from ten to forty grains.

The internal administration of tar is also stated to be beneficial when other remedies fail, but it is by no means a drug to be relied upon.

The local treatment of psoriasis is most important, but though the employment of it without any internal remedy does remove the external appearance of the disease, a real cure is not effected on account of its liability to return. Both modes of treatment should, therefore, be adopted at the same time, and the internal should be continued for a considerable period after the apparent cure.

When the inflammation is excessive the continuous application of cold water is of great benefit in removing the scales and limiting their production.

This may be carried out by means of baths or by local cold packing; the former should be done thoroughly by immersion of the whole body or one limb for many hours at a time.

Before applying local remedies it is necessary first to endeavour to remove the scales. This is best carried out by means of soft soap, and so effectual is this plan sometimes that no further application is required.

Of local remedies those of a stimulating character are the most suitable, such as preparations of tar. The huile de cade, or common tar itself, or better still the liquor carbonis detergens, ought to be tried, but no drug has proved so successful in such a large proportion of cases as chrysophanic acid, which may be used in the form of an ointment consisting of ten to thirty grains of the acid to one ounce of vaseline or lard. Chrysophanic acid is the active principle of Goa powder, the Indian remedy for ringworm, and was first recommended in psoriasis by Mr. Balmanno Squire. The chief objection to this drug is the amount of irritation it produces, not so much in the patch to which it has been applied, but in the neighbouring skin. Sometimes this irritation is very severe, when the use of the remedy should be immediately suspended.

PITYRIASIS.

Definition.—Pityriasis is a chronic squamous disease of the skin, in which the scales are branny and are seated on a non-infiltrated surface.

Symptoms.—The eruption consists of the production of a quantity of fine scales, which are continually being shed and reproduced. The skin of the affected part may be slightly red, but there is no effusion into or thickening of the epidermic layer. There is but slight itching of the part, and, unless the skin be delicate, excoriations rarely result from scratching. Any portion of the body may be affected with pityriasis, but the most common sites are the hairy parts, more particularly the scalp. The ordinary condition, known as pityriasis capitis, has been shown by Hebra to be due to an increased secretion of the sebaceous glands, and is in no sense of the word a pityriasis.

Diagnosis.—Pityriasis may be confounded with—

1. Psoriasis see (p. 149).
2. Tinea tonsurans. The only certain mode of diagnosis is by the use of the microscope, which shows the characteristic fungus elements in tinea; in addition, to the naked eye the hair is seen to be broken off short, and is easily extracted.

Prognosis.—Pityriasis is a chronic and often intractable disease, but is never attended with any serious result.

Treatment.—It is usually treated locally by the application of alkaline lotions. The best are carbonate of potash, ʒj to the half-pint; or liquor potassæ, ʒij to ℥viij of water. Ointments containing either a little sulphur or mercury, or both combined, are useful. In very protracted cases arsenic may be tried.

CHAPTER XIV.

Class I.—EXUDATIONES—*continued.*

6. *PHLEGMONOUS AND ULCERATIVE GROUP.*

Furunculus—Anthrax—Delhi Boil—Ulcers.

FURUNCULUS—BOIL.

Definition.—A boil is an acute localised inflammation of
the true skin, which usually terminates in necrosis and discharge by suppuration of a central portion or 'core.'

Symptoms.—The ordinary follicular boil begins as a small
hard, painful spot in the true skin, which soon becomes red on
the surface. Inflammatory swelling, heat, and pain rapidly
occur, and in the course of a day or two a small subconical
elevation, which throbs and is acutely sensitive, is produced.
A minute yellow spot next appears at the apex of the swelling,
the cuticle thins and ruptures, and pus is gradually discharged
from a small orifice. As the orifice enlarges, within it is seen
a greyish or yellow slough, called the 'core.' This becomes
loosened and finally cast off, together with shreddy pus; and as
the inflammatory redness and swelling subside, the little cavity
fills up with granulations and heals, leaving a slightly depressed, often pigmented scar.

In the 'blind' or subcutaneous boil the starting-point is
in the deeper layers of the cutis; the tumour is therefore less
prominent, and pus is slower in reaching the surface. The process is, however, the same in both varieties.

Boils are most frequently excited by local irritants, such as
the undue use of hydropathic bandages and poultices, or from
post-mortem virus, &c.; but in certain states of the system

·there appears to be a special predisposition to their occurrence. Persons suffering from diabetes or convalescent from acute diseases, especially enteric fever, seem specially liable to them. Though single boils cause little or no disturbance of the general system, yet when they are numerous and extensive, and occur in weakly and irritable individuals, there may be considerable fever.

Diagnosis.—The circumscribed, painful swelling, going on to suppuration with the discharge of a 'core,' cannot well be mistaken for any other skin affection.

Prognosis.—The course of a boil is usually towards recovery after suppuration has set in, but occasionally it may disappear spontaneously, or under treatment, without breaking. They are prone to recur, and successive crops may last for weeks.

Morbid Anatomy.—This is included under Anthrax.

Treatment.—In the early stage mercury with belladonna and glycerine, or the application of belladonna or soap plaister, is said to check the development of a boil. When more advanced, frequent poulticing, to relieve pain and to promote the discharge and separation of the sloughs, is the proper treatment. Yeast, in doses of a tablespoonful two or three times daily, is said to be of use in preventing fresh attacks; but the most appropriate internal remedies are quinine and iron or ammonia and bark. The diet should be generous and liberal, with a fair amount of beer and good port wine; and, in addition, change of air may be recommended.

ANTHRAX—CARBUNCLE.

Definition.—An acute localised inflammation of the true skin, differing from that in furunculus by the multiplicity of the cores and by the liability of the intervening skin and the subjacent tissues to slough. The constitutional symptoms are usually severe.

Symptoms.—Carbuncle begins as a flattened, slightly elevated swelling of the true skin, slightly red in colour, and

attended with severe pain and marked fever. Usually there are
several points of intense inflammation, that lead to necrosis of
the tissues and the formation of ' cores.' Considerable inflammatory infiltration surrounds the little nodule. As in a boil,
suppuration soon commences; but, as the cores usually form
only the superficial indications of more extensive subcutaneous
sloughs, it has to continue a long time before they are separated, during which lymphangitis, cellulitis, and septic absorption, giving rise to pyæmia, may occur.

Carbuncles appear most frequently on the nape of the neck,
buttocks, and external surfaces of the limbs; they occasionally
arise on the face and lips, in which situations the liability to
phlebitis and fatal septicæmia is very great. They are usually
solitary, but sometimes are multiple, and not infrequently a
succession of them appears in different parts of the body.

Diagnosis.—Carbuncle can only be mistaken for a collection
of boils which have become confluent. The more intense pain
and constitutional symptoms, the more extensive subcutaneous
necrosis, and the greater proneness to sloughing of the skin
will serve to distinguish it.

Prognosis.—Carbuncle, always an affection of serious import, is especially grave in those suffering from exhausting
diseases or in a cachectic condition, however produced. The
intense pain, causing sleeplessness, and the nervous exhaustion,
the severe fever, the prolonged suppuration, with the special
liability to septicæmia, in carbuncle of the face and lip, are all
elements which intensify the danger in proportion as they are
well marked.

Morbid Anatomy.—Both of these affections, boil and carbuncle, may be considered together, the essential feature being
the formation of necrosed masses of tissue, which are solitary
in the former and form the ' core.' A carbuncle containing
several ' cores' may be considered anatomically as formed by
the confluence of several boils. The morbid anatomy has not
been thoroughly made out; it is stated, however, that there
is an acute inflammation either in the connective tissue

passing from the base of a hair follicle down into the subcutaneous fatty tissue, or around one or more sebaceous glands,
as the primary phenomenon. The hyperæmia and abundant
exudation of plasma into the loose subcutaneous tissue form
the large swelling round the central spot. The accumulation
of cells and plasma being excessive, the blood supply is either
cut off from the central core, or the vessels round become
thrombosed, and in consequence the mass dies. A 'line of
demarcation' soon forms, and the 'core' becomes loose and can
be removed.

In anthrax the process is the same; the 'cores,' however,
are multiple, there is much more œdema of the cellular tissue,
and the intensity of the inflammation may cut off the blood
supply from the intervening tissue, causing a greyish slough or
black gangrenous mass.

Treatment.—An abundant, nutritious, and easily digested
diet, with stimulants in proportion as the patient is depressed
or debilitated, are essential parts of the general treatment.
Iron and quinine, or ammonia and bark, as for boils, should be
given. As measures of local treatment the free crucial incision,
the subcutaneous incision of the nodule, and cauterisation with
potassa fusa, have been advised and practised. In the early
stages Hebra recommends the application of cold, by means of
ice bladders, to check the extension of inflammation and subsequent suppuration. Poultices and warm poppy fomentations,
with some antiseptic, such as carbolic acid or thymol, to lessen
the risk of septic absorption and to promote the separation of the
sloughs, are undoubtedly useful. These measures are probably
quite as efficacious as the more active treatment mentioned
above.

DELHI BOIL.

Definition.—A chronic endemic disease met with in India,
characterised by the production of a small flattened nodule,
which undergoes slow ulceration and heals with loss of substance, leaving a whitish, depressed scar.

Symptoms.—Delhi boil is said to begin as a small reddish spot with a central papule, gradually enlarging to form a smooth, reddish-brown, flattened nodule, which then begins to desquamate and ulcerate. Yellowish white points, which are the altered hair and gland follicles, soon become covered with a thin scab, under which suppuration slowly goes on. An indolent sore with hard edges and base of flabby granulations is present under the scab. After lasting two or three months the sore usually begins to heal, and leaves a whitish, irregular scar.

The disease attacks the exposed parts of the body, and does not seem materially to affect the general health. It is said to be communicable by inoculation.

Morbid Anatomy.—This is described as follows. Microscopic examination of the papule before ulceration has begun shows the connective tissue of the corium infiltrated with masses of cells, oval or roundish in shape, yellowish brown, and with one or more nuclei. The glands and papillæ appear to be destroyed by this growth, and the hair follicles become enlarged, while here and there these cystic dilatations are observed in the hairs themselves. After ulceration has commenced, in the purulent discharge pigmented bodies, resembling the ova of distomata, are said sometimes to occur.

Treatment.—Local treatment only is necessary, consisting in the thorough application of strong nitric acid if the nodule be in an early stage, or of potassa fusa if an ulcer have formed, which converts the disease into a simple ulcer that soon heals.

ULCERS.

The following brief account of ulcers and their treatment has been contributed by Mr. Edmund Owen :—

An ulcer is well defined as being a solution of continuity with loss of substance. The common cause of ulceration of the skin is suppuration in the dermal connective tissue. The collecting pus, in its escape to the surface, destroys the superimposed dermal layer; and the epidermis, being thus deprived of its nutritive supply, dies and is shed.

Now, whatever conditions interfere with the nutrition of the skin necessarily predispose to the formation of ulcers. Thus when the function of the veins of the leg becomes impaired from a failure of the valves to check the downward fall of the blood, stagnation in, or rather congestion of, the cutaneous capillaries results, and from the distended vessels the serum oozes, so that the tissues become œdematous, pitting on pressure.

In this sodden and unhealthy skin a comparatively slight irritation, or trivial injury, is frequently attended by lesions, troublesome out of all proportion. And thus the chafing of a badly-fitting boot, or the fretting of a dirty or rough stocking, or a knock against a stair, may determine the formation of an ulcer, which will persistently refuse to yield to ordinary therapeutic measures.

As a rule varicose ulcers are associated with eczema, an attack of eczema often preceding and determining their onset.

Common sense, with a little practice, will soon enable the student to select with great promptness the adjectives best describing the varicose ulcer, but the term 'chronic' only too often denotes its chief characteristic.

The following is a list of the different kinds of ulcers usually met with :—

The *healthy* ulcer, which is circular and is generally covered by a little thick pus; the granulations red and even with the surface of the part; the edge of the sore is covered by a slightly depressed, bluish-white film of new epidermis, which gradually loses itself in sound tissue. The treatment, whatever it may be, is evidently well chosen, for the sore is healing.

The *weak* ulcer is covered by large and pale granulations, which are heaped up on the surface but are painless. The local treatment best adapted will be rest, aided by the pressure of a pad of dry lint and a bandage or strapping. Stimulating lotions may be of use, also resinous and other ointments. A change of application is often attended with such good results that the weak ulcer is converted into one of the preceding class.

The *indolent* ulcer is grey and glazed, and is surrounded by an unyielding mass of tissue, which has been rendered thick and discoloured from long-continued congestion. The discharge is thin, and often of a most foul odour.

Blistering fluid applied around the margin may sometimes effect much good by causing absorption of plastic deposit; but the poor and ill-fed can rarely submit to such treatment as out-patients. With in-patients two semi-elliptical incisions on the side of the sore will relieve much tension and promote a healthy condition.

The *inflamed* ulcer is recognised by placing over it, but not in contact with its raw and painful surface, the palm of the hand. The parts around are livid, hot, and tense. Poulticing affords great relief by diminishing the heat and pain.

The *phagedœnic* or *gangrenous* ulcer is, as the former term implies, a sore which extends by eating its way into the neigh-bouring skin. It shows no attempt at healing; on the con-trary, the discharge is thin and bloody, and the surrounding parts are livid and swollen.

Opium given internally with quinine and acid; poultices and cleansing lotions; and the hot leg-bath will be required.

The *irritable* ulcer is to be distinguished from the in-flamed ulcer by the absence of heat when the hand is held over it, as well as by the watery nature of the fluid thrown off from its surface. It is exceedingly painful, and its essen-tial pathological character depends, according to Hilton, on the exposure of a nerve upon its surface. The exquisitely tender spot is to be made out by searching over the granula-tions with a probe; the treatment will consist in the division of the twig above the spot indicated by the examination. Opium and tonics may be required.

Although the leg and ankle are the most frequent seats of ulcers, on account of the unfavourable influence with which the force of gravity continually acts upon the venous blood, still it is hardly necessary to remark that there may be other than varicose ulcers even on the surface of the lower extremity. Any part of the body may be the seat of an ulceration which is the result of the destructive influence of neoplastic deposits. Thus are begotten the *tubercular*, the *lupoid*, and the *syphilitic* ulcers.

But to give a description of all these varieties of sore would be to write an essay on pathology, which, in the small space which can be devoted to the subject, is manifestly impossible. So we must content ourselves by concluding with a few general remarks which may be found of service to the student in his early practice.

First, then, when ulcers are found in regions where one is not accustomed to see them, as upon the knee, calf, thigh, trunk, arm, or face, they are not unfrequently of syphilitic origin.

Of course the integument of these areas may be attacked by ulcers which are not the result of syphilis. But if the sores are multiple, clean-cut, with rounded or crescentic margins, and appearing in successive crops, there is quite enough to justify the suspicion of the student, and even, it may be, to induce him to commence the treatment of the patient with the internal adminis- tration of iodide of potassium in full doses. But we will venture here to offer him two cautions—firstly, not to place too much faith in what is known as a 'coppery stain' about an ulcer; and, secondly, not to conclude that, because an ulcer has healed whilst the iodide is being taken, therefore the sore was the result of a breaking down of a deposit left as the result of syphilitic infection.

A last word concerning the treatment of those number- less ulcers which are the result of dilated veins. They occur chiefly in laundresses, ironers, ostlers, and others who stand much during the day, and who drink freely, whether of tea or beer. Rest is more easily enjoined than enforced; but the amount of vascular fulness may be diminished by regulating

M

the amount of fluid absorbed. The veins require support; but this cannot often be obtained in the shape of the costly elastic stocking, nor, if there be eczema present, could that useful aid be tolerated, for the moisture from the vesicular eruption would soon render the webbing hard, irritating, and worse than useless.

Martin's indiarubber bandages are useful in some cases, but their application requires more care and manipulative skill than these patients usually possess, whilst their cost often puts them beyond the reach of most of these sufferers. Considerable success may be obtained by applying a piece of strapping firmly, but not too tightly, around the limb, *above* the ulcer and below the dilated veins, leaving the sore exposed for the application of lotions or ointments. Theory might perhaps suggest that such a method of treatment is unscientific, as it would offer another barrier to the easy return of the venous stream. But practice shows that the strapping so applied generally affords the greatest comfort by cutting off the weight of the downward-pressing column of venous blood, in the same way that the application of a truss affords relief in a bad case of varicocele. The strapping is best applied by the patient before he gets out of bed in the morning; its use may be dispensed with at night. In some cases of varicose eczema also the wearing of a garter below the knee affords great relief.

163

CHAPTER XV.

Class II.—Vascular Affections.

Hyperæmia—Anæmia—Hæmorrhages of the Skin—Purpura simplex,
papulosa, rheumatica, hæmorrhagica—Scorbutus—Hæmatidrosis.

In the class of Vascular Affections of the Skin the subdivisions
Hyperæmia, Anæmia, and Hæmorrhages are included.

In themselves the two first are of slight importance and do
not endanger life; but as the manifestations or symptoms of
graver conditions, or as the early stages of further changes in
the skin, they require a more complete description. Cutaneous
hæmorrhages are similarly of slight moment if not symptomatic
of variola, scarlatina, typhus, &c., and of the so-called purpura
hæmorrhagica, which is more properly a general vascular disease
than one of the skin.

HYPERÆMIA.

The hyperæmic affections, characterised in general by an
undue injection of blood into the capillaries, small veins, and
arterioles of the superficial layer of the skin, fall conveniently
into the two subdivisions of active and passive.

In the former of these the skin has usually a brighter red
colour, and the appearance is accompanied by a feeling of irritation, as of burning or itching, by moderate swelling, and sometimes by slight elevation of temperature; while in the latter
the hue is more livid, the temperature lowered or only normal,
and a feeling is experienced of numbness or even anæsthesia.
The division between these two forms is merely one of conveni-
ence, as the active hyperæmia may culminate in the passive (con-

M 2

gestion), or they may be present side by side on the same portion
of skin, as in thrombosis or embolism, when the central part is
in a state of congestion and the marginal in one of active
hyperæmia.

Active Hyperæmia as defined presents varieties which may
be classed under the two headings of—

1. Traumatic, excited by irritants.

2. Symptomatic, arising in the course of other diseases,
probably under the influence of reflex irritation of the nervous
system.

The former are usually called erythemata, a term to which
a special meaning has been already assigned (p. 99), and, as they
are characterised chiefly by an increased vascularity, with little
or no exudation, the more suitable name of hyperæmia will here
be used.

a. Hyperæmia (erythema) *mechanica* arises on portions of
skin exposed to undue pressure, rubbing, or scratching. It is
usually transient, but if the irritant be repeatedly in action the
skin is prone to become the seat of congestion or of inflammatory
change, and the eruptions of exanthemata appear upon it with
special brightness.

b. Hyperæmia calorica arises on parts exposed to the sun's
rays, or to winds, as a diffuse bright-red discoloration, which in
time becomes darker and usually ends in brownish pigmentation
and slight desquamation. Transient degrees of heat, and either
warm or cold baths, excite a fugitive hyperæmia.

c. Hyperæmia ab acribus seu venenata is produced by the
slight action of chemical irritants, the juice of certain plants,
mustard, &c., and readily developes into exudation and inflammation if the cause be prolonged.

Symptomatic Hyperæmia may be excited by physical causes,
such as anger, shame, &c.—*i.e.* in the form of a blush or of a
more diffuse and slighter injection—or it may arise in the course
of dentition or gastric disturbances in infancy, when it has
been termed erythema, roseola infantilis, strophulus, &c., or

vaccinia, variola, enteric fever, cholera, rheumatism, and other diseases, when it has been variously named erythema or roseola vaccinia, &c.

Passive Hyperæmia may be either general, under the influence of heart or lung disease, causing mechanical congestion, or local, from pressure on the veins or deficient arterial *vis a tergo*. The two latter, which have been termed livedo mechanica and livedo calorica respectively by Hebra, will now be described.

Livedo mechanica, arising under the influence of pressure from tight clothes, garters, varicose veins, &c., appears as a purplish red, bluish, or greyish black discoloration of the skin, disappearing under pressure, with slight swelling if there be no œdema. When the cause is removed it gradually subsides.

Livedo calorica is the name applied to the bluish-red or purplish tint seen on the nose, ears, &c., of persons exposed to the cold, and to the dark lines about half or three-quarters of an inch wide which form serpentine figures on the extremities and trunk. The latter are chiefly visible on the extremities, and, but less obviously, on the trunk, and though fading on pressure, disappear only when the patient is warm. Occasionally in the midst of the purplish background vermilion-red patches are observable, varying in size from $\frac{1}{8}$ to $\frac{1}{3}$ of an inch, and sometimes surrounded by a pale zone.

If the action of cold be prolonged, it may in weakly, chlorotic persons give rise not only to congestion, but to exudation and an eczematous condition to which the name chilblain has been applied.

Morbid Anatomy.—The active hyperæmiæ leave little or no traces for examination after death beyond slight pigmentation of the rete cells. The experiments of Auspitz lead him to a very probable explanation of the persistence after removing the ligature of the brown pigmentation subsequently left by the vermilion-coloured spots noticed in passive hyperæmia. He ascribes it to the admixture with the transuded serum in the tissue of red corpuscles, which subsequently give rise to hæmatoidin crystals and yellow or brown pigment. The pale streaks are due to the shutting off from the circulation of certain tracts of vessels which are empty or contain only clear serum, as in embolism, &c.

ANÆMIA.

Anæmia of the skin may be general, as in chlorosis, after loss of blood, exhausting discharges, &c. ; or local, under the influence of cold, undue action of local vasomotor nerves, pressure, &c.

It is of importance only so far as it modifies the appearances of eruptions, and produces apparent retrogression in such as are characterised by hyperæmia. Thus the exanthems of scarlatina and measles may fade if exposed to cold, or an old psoriasis be lost sight of after severe hæmorrhage, only to reappear as the former vascularity of the skin returns.

Treatment.—The application of cold water, spirit lotion, or lotio carbonis detergens, to relieve the burning and itching in active hyperæmia, is all that is necessary.

HÆMORRHAGES OF THE SKIN.

A. Traumatic . . . From wounds, bruises.

B. Symptomatic . . {
  1. Purpura { Simplex / Papulosa / Rheumatica / Hæmorrhagica
  2. Scorbutus
  3. Hæmatidrosis
}

Extravasations of blood in the skin take the form of—

1. *Petechiæ*—round or irregular, bright or livid red spots, not raised, varying from $\frac{1}{16}$ to $\frac{1}{2}$ an inch in size, appearing as if splashed on the skin.

2. *Vibices*—long streaks, either branching or parallel to one another.

3. *Ecchymoses*—dark-red irregular patches, varying in diameter from 1 to 3 inches.

They do not fade on pressure, but undergo a series of

changes from red to brown, greenish, and yellow before they disappear.

A. *Traumatic.*—The ordinary appearances of a bruise, or ecchymosis, produced, for instance, by a blow on the skin, and the minute petechiæ due to flea or bug bites, are familiar to everyone.

B. *Symptomatic.*

PURPURA.

Definition.—Extravasations of blood occurring as puncta, petechiæ, vibices, or ecchymoses, either spontaneously or in the course of various diseases.

Symptoms.—The following varieties have been described :—

a. Purpura simplex consists in the occurrence of numerous petechiæ, or vibices, irregularly scattered over the body, usually most markedly on the legs, where there is a tendency to symmetry of the eruption. The disease is said to occur in debilitated persons, but is attended by little or no subjective trouble, and is not dangerous to life. When small papules appear between the hæmorrhages the affection is. termed *purpura papulosa.*

b. Pupura rheumatica, or *Peliosis rheumatica,* first described as a separate disease under the latter name by Schönlein, is characterised by rheumatic pains in and about the joints, together with an appearance of a rash, which is at first erythematous but soon becomes hæmorrhagic. Though provisionally classed with purpura, it ought rather to be considered a variety of erythema papulatum or nodosum, with which, according to Bazin and others, it is identical. According to Hebra it arises with dragging pains in the joints and some fever, followed in a few days by the eruption near the joints, or more especially on the abdomen and breast. The spots, round and flat, are only slightly raised, gradually fade, with the usual changes of colour, and disappear, without desquamation, in a week.

The disease usually attacks strong and healthy persons between the ages of twenty and thirty, and more frequently males than females. It has never been seen in children or aged persons.

c. Purpura hæmorrhagica is a severe constitutional variety, in which the cutaneous extravasations are abundant and large, and accompanied by hæmorrhages into various organs and from mucous surfaces. Marked anæmia and asthenia are induced by the severe losses of blood, and death is not an infrequent result.

The so-called purpura fibrilis is usually only a purpuric rash that appears in the course of one of the acute infectious diseases.

Diagnosis.—A petechial rash, not occurring in the course of one of the exanthemata, may be mistaken for—

1. Flea bites. 2. Scurvy.

Flea bites are most abundant where the folds of the clothes are thick, as on the neck, wrists, waist, and ankles; while purpura affects the lower limbs pre-eminently, and has no special predilection for other sites. It is also hæmorrhagic from the beginning, and does not appear as a roseolar spot, or wheal, with a central red dot.

The following table will show the points of difference from scurvy :—

SCURVY.	PURPURA.
1. Is due to privation from vegetables and to depressing circumstances, and is cured by lime juice and fruit.	1. Is not produced by want of vegetables, and lime juice has no influence on its course.
2. Affects usually many persons at the same time.	2. Occurs sporadically.
3. The gums become spongy, the teeth loose, and painful subcutaneous ecchymoses, prone to suppuration, may occur.	3. No affection of gums or painful ecchymoses.
4. Is attended with great prostration and a peculiar dusky pallor of skin.	4. Prostration only proportionate to loss of blood; skin anæmic.
5. Death occurs rarely from hæmorrhage, usually from serous effusions or septicæmia.	5. Death results from asthenia or syncope, the result of hæmorrhage.

Prognosis.—Purpura simplex and rheumatica are affections of slight gravity, and as a rule tend towards spontaneous recovery. Purpura hæmorrhagica is serious in proportion to the amount of internal bleeding; it often resists treatment, and proves fatal by anæmia and exhaustion or syncope.

Morbid Anatomy.—The skin, after death, of a person who during life has had purpura shows—

1. Recent hæmorrhagic spots in the form of subarticular or interstitial puncta, or striæ of a dark purplish colour.

2. Small crusts of dark colour, due to the drying up of the petechiæ.

3. Brownish or yellowish stains, marking the position of former hæmorrhages of which the fluid portions have become absorbed and the blood corpuscles more or less altered.

In a section of a recent petechial spot, either in the fresh condition or after hardening, the effusion of blood is seen to be mainly limited to the papillary layer of the corium and the overlying rete Malpighii. On microscopic examination blood corpuscles, the majority of which are more or less broken down, are seen surrounding the hair follicles, having apparently proceeded from the capillary network round the latter. Should the effusions take the form of vibices, the blood corpuscles are found in and around the papillæ of the corium and in the rete, raising the horny layers of the epidermis as in a vesicle.

Microscopic examination of the older spots shows the blood corpuscles broken down and converted into pigment, reddish-brown masses and granules of which are found lying in the meshes of the connective tissue of the corium, and sometimes staining the branched cells a brownish-yellow colour.

In the majority of cases of purpura simplex in which a microscopic examination of the blood capillaries has been made, no obvious morbid changes have been found.

Dr. Wilson Fox described albuminoid or lardaceous changes in the capillaries in the vicinity of purpuric spots as traceable in some cases, and in the cutaneous hæmorrhages occurring in certain instances of phosphorus poisoning acute fatty degeneration has been found in the arterioles and capillaries, to the rupture of which the extravasations are ascribed.

Where no alteration of the capillaries has taken place the escape of the red corpuscles is supposed to be due to simple diapedesis, the resistance of the capillary walls being so diminished as to allow the passage through them of red corpuscles when, from any slight exertion, as in standing, strain is thrown upon them.

Treatment.—In the milder forms of purpura, rest in bed, nutritious diet, and tonics are all that is needed.

In purpura hæmorrhagica various drugs, chiefly metallic astringents and those which act on the blood vessels, have been used; of these, tinctura ferri perchloridi, in doses of xx to xxx drops three times a day, either alone or with ergot and digitalis, gives the best results.

SCORBUTUS—SCURVY.

Definition.—Scurvy is a general disease of the body characterised by progressive anæmia, severe mental prostration and asthenia, impairment of nutrition and a tendency to the occurrence of hæmorrhages from mucous membranes and into the skin, muscles, and viscera. It is due to privation from, or an insufficient supply of, fresh vegetable food.

Symptoms.—The patient presents at first a dirty, pallid, or earthy-looking complexion, accompanied by languor and *malaise*, mental apathy and depression, and rheumatic pains in the back and the muscles of the limbs. The gums swell, forming deep red spongy masses round the teeth, which are prone to bleed and ulcerate, giving great fœtor to the breath. The teeth may loosen and drop out. Petechiæ appear at first on the lower limbs, followed by ecchymoses and subcutaneous extravasations, which spontaneously, or on slight irritation or injury, are liable to suppurate and give rise to unhealthy, painful, bleeding ulcers. Progressive anæmia, sudden syncope on slight exertion, sanguineous effusions into the pleura and pericardium, gangrene of the lungs, or diarrhœa, may lead to a fatal result.

Diagnosis.—From purpura (see p. 168).

Prognosis.—It is serious and often fatal if untreated. Death results most frequently from asthenia or sudden syncope. Cases of moderate severity almost always recover if fresh vegetables be added to the dietary.

Morbid Anatomy.—The cutaneous changes resemble those met with in purpura, already described.

Treatment.—The essential point in the treatment is the restoration to the diet of vegetable food in the form of fruits, green vegetables, turnips, carrots, onions, lemon or lime juice.

The gum affection should be treated by antiseptic and astringent washes. The tendency to syncope should be averted by rest in bed, stimulants, and digitalis.

HÆMATIDROSIS.

Hæmatidrosis, or 'bloody sweat,' is an affection of rare occurrence. It is a hæmorrhage on the surface of the skin in parts where the cuticle is thin and delicate, and it is produced by rupture of capillaries in the plexus round the mouths of the sweat ducts.

The 'stigmata' on the forehead, hands, and feet, stated to occur in the persons of religious fanatics, have proved in most cases, when submitted to a careful scientific examination, to be fictitious.

CHAPTER XVI.

Class III.—NEUROSES.

Zoster—Cheiro-pompholyx—Pruritus—Dystrophia cutis.

ZOSTER—HERPES ZOSTER—SHINGLES.

Definition.—Zoster is a disease of acute and typical course and benign nature, characterised by the eruption of groups of vesicles or erythematous papules, which correspond in situation with the peripheral distribution of a cutaneous nerve—usually on one side of the body—and are produced through the influence of irritative lesions of the nervous system.

Following the classification of Hebra, zoster is divided into the following varieties :—

1. Zoster capillitii.
2. Zoster faciei.
3. Zoster nuchæ et colli { occipito-collaris. cervico-subclavicularis.
4. Zoster cervico-brachialis.
5. Zoster pectoralis.
6. Zoster abdominalis.
7. Zoster femoralis.

Symptoms.—Usually after a few days, sometimes a few weeks, of neuralgic pains, either over the whole region which becomes subsequently affected, or at certain fixed spots corresponding with points of division or emergence from the deeper tissues of cutaneous nerves, the eruption appears suddenly. It consists of an efflorescence of bright red papules, about the size of millet seeds, on an erythematous surface, and is accompanied usually by a burning sensation. Within a few hours, or in a day or two, the papules become vesicles, from the size of a pin's head to that of a pea, filled with a clear serous fluid; they are either quite isolated or closely aggregated, and sometimes by confluence form an irregular bulla. Successive crops of vesicles may prolong the eruptive stage for a week, but each series has all its vesicles at the same stage of development; thus one group may be papular, another vesicular, and a third already desiccated.

After a day or two the contents of the vesicles become opaque and purulent; they then dry up, forming yellow scabs, which usually, about a fortnight after the onset of the affection, fall off, leaving reddish-brown stained patches. Successive efflorescences may, however, prolong the total duration of the disease to three or four weeks, but they always appear upon adjacent portions of skin, *never* on that implicated by the first eruption. The vesicles may be few in number, and confined to a circumscribed area, or closely aggregated along the whole course of a nerve; in the latter case the pain and constitutional symptoms are somewhat severe, and the duration of the attack more prolonged.

As zoster is not usually a fatal disease, cases in which the cause has been ascertained by autopsy are rare. Bärensprung, Charcot, Wagner, Kaposi, and others have found as the most frequent cause hæmorrhage and inflammation of the intervertebral or Gasserian ganglia.

New growths, carcinomatous, tubercular, or purulent collections, causing irritation of the adjacent nerve-trunks or ganglia; traumatic lesions, causing irritation of the peripheral sensory or mixed nerves and meningitis; caries of the vertebræ or locomotor ataxy, causing irritation of the posterior roots—are frequently attended with eruptions of zoster. It has also been noticed after poisoning with carbonic oxide gas, and occasionally during the administration of arsenic (Hutchinson). Hebra and Kaposi, on whose descriptions this account is mainly based, consider as abnormal the following variations in the course and consequences of zoster :—

1. Cases in which some part or all of the eruption remains papular and aborts or forms bullæ or pustules, the latter causing destruction of the dermis and giving rise to lasting cicatrices.

2. Cases in which blood appears in the contents of the vesicles, or hæmorrhagic infiltration of their bases occurs. In the latter the vesicles burst, the infiltrated tissue of their bases slowly necroses, and extremely painful ulcers, which take weeks or months to heal, and which leave permanent scars, are produced.

3. Cases in which neuralgia does not abate with the efflorescence, but persists during and long after the eruption. This is rare in the young, more common in the aged.

4. Cases where muscular atrophy, anæsthesia, alopecia, or loss of teeth or atrophy of the alveolar process occurs after the zoster.

5. Bilateral symmetrical zoster.

Zoster usually occurs but once in a lifetime; it rarely passes the middle line before or behind, and then only slightly; it appears at all ages and in both sexes; it affects either side of the body indifferently, being, according to statistics, slightly more common on the right. The groups of vesicles formed are, according to Hebra, always nearest the nervous centres, the subsequent crops lying more towards the periphery of the corresponding nerves.

1. *Zoster capillitii*, best seen in bald persons, occurs on the scalp in the peripheral distribution of the supra-orbital and great occipital nerves, and sometimes forms an arch over one parietal bone, terminating near the coronal suture.

2. *Zoster faciei* presents the greatest variety of appearances. Groups of vesicles, limited accurately by the middle line, may appear on the forehead along the course of the supra-orbital nerve; at the inner angle of the orbit and root of the nose along the supra-trochlear; on the cheek, ala nasi, and lower eyelid along the infra-orbital; and in the mouth, palate, and pharynx from implication of the palatine branches of the superior maxillary. Vesicles may appear on the gums, associated with violent toothache, loosening and loss of the teeth, and atrophy of the

alveolar process when the superior dental is affected. The eruption may also appear in the region of the auriculo-temporal, on the temple, pinna and meatus of the ear, on the chin, the mental branch, and on the side of the tongue in the course of the lingual. When the whole region of distribution of the ophthalmic branch of the fifth nerve is affected, in addition to the zoster frontalis there are vesicles, very often hæmorrhagic, on the nose and nasal mucous membrane, from affection of the infratrochlear and ethmoidal twigs, vesicles on the temple and malar prominence, from the zygomatic and lachrymal branches, and conjunctivitis, corneal ulcers, and iritis, from affection of the long root of the lenticular ganglion. Ophthalmitis, thrombosis of the ophthalmic vein, septicæmia, and death may thus result from zoster ophthalmicus.

3. *Zoster nuchæ et colli.*—The variety occipito-collaris presents vesicles on the back of the neck from the great and small occipital nerves, on the posterior surface of the pinna and lobule (great auricular), and on the side of the neck and beneath the chin. The variety cervico-subclavicularis occurs in the region of distribution of the ascending and descending cutaneous branches of the cervical plexus, on the region of the neck below the scalp back as far as the shoulder and downwards as far as the skin between the clavicle and nipple.

4. *Zoster cervico-brachialis* affects the brachial plexus, and presents groups of vesicles on both sides of the arm and forearm as far as the little finger, and on the second and third intercostal spaces as far as the sternum.

5. *Zoster pectoralis* occurs—

a. As a continuous band of vesicles, occupying one to three intercostal spaces, running from the spine to the sternum; to this the terms *zona* and *shingles* were originally applied. The vesicles not unfrequently coalesce, and are sometimes hæmorrhagic; in the latter case the pain is excessive.

b. As patches of vesicles, one usually near the spine, corresponding to the hinder branches of the dorsal nerve; one on the side of the thorax, where the twig of the intercostal nerve penetrates the muscles, and a third near the sternum, at the termination of the nerve. The spinal and sternal groups may pass the middle line about half an inch, and even in bilateral zoster the groups never coalesce to form a complete girdle, as the ends overlap. One group only may be present.

The intense pain in the side and the dyspnœa may sometimes lead to a suspicion of pleurisy.

6. *Zoster femoralis* presents groups of vesicles, appearing usually first on the buttock, to which region they may be confined, or on the front or on the back of the thigh, and they may extend downwards to the ham or calf. On the penis *zoster pudentalis*, from affections of the pudic nerve, may occur, but is sharply restricted to one side of the organ (Kaposi).

Diagnosis.—The sudden appearance, usually preceded by neuralgic pain of a group of vesicles situated on the peripheral distribution of a cutaneous nerve, and the course of the affection, are sufficient, even in abortive cases, to distinguish zoster from any other vesicular disease of the skin.

Prognosis.—Zoster is a benign disease. An extensive efflorescence of the hæmorrhagic form, with slow-healing, painful ulcers or severe neuralgia, may wear out an aged, weakly person, but death rarely results except from some intercurrent malady.

Morbid Anatomy.—In the intervertebral ganglia undue vascularity of the surrounding fatty tissue of the ganglion itself and intracapsular hæmorrhages have been found. Under the microscope the capillaries of the ganglion are found loaded with blood, the ganglion cells separated and destroyed by hæmorrhage, and sometimes surrounded inside their capsules, and numerous leucocytes are scattered throughout the tissue. When due to affections of the peripheral nerves, at a distance from the ganglion, the condition is usually one of subacute neuritis. The nerve is greyish, slightly injected, thickened, adherent to its sheath and adjacent parts, and on microscopic examination an excess of spindle cells are found in it, causing granular degeneration of the medullary sheath and the axis cylinders. The vesicles present no essential difference from those of herpes febrilis or eczema. The acute neuritis of the peripheral nerves found by Haight near the vesicles resembles that met with in many other inflammations of the corium, and is not peculiar to zoster.

Treatment.—No internal or local remedies have yet proved of the slightest use in cutting short an attack of zoster; all that remains to be done, therefore, is to palliate the severity of the symptoms, and to let the disease run its natural course, avoiding, as worse than useless, any attempt, by cauterisation or otherwise, to check the formation of the vesicles. Dusting with powder, and covering with cotton wool and a bandage to prevent the clothes rubbing the vesicles, and, if ulcers form, dressing in the usual way, is all that is needed locally. Should the pain be intense, narcotics by the mouth, or better still hypodermically, ought to be used. The subsequent neuralgia, which is often severe in the aged, is best treated by quinine and arsenic in full doses, and by the repeated application of the continuous current.

CHEIRO-POMPHOLYX (*Hutchinson*).

Definition.—A disease of the skin characterised by the appearance of small clear vesicles or bullæ on the hands, and sometimes on the feet, usually symmetrical, running a short course, and liable to constant relapses.

Symptoms.—The disease, in its milder forms, is not very uncommon, but the more severe cases, in which large bullæ are produced, are extremely rare.

In persons of nervous temperament, when out of health or worried and depressed, the disease begins by burning and itching between and along the sides of the fingers, followed in a few hours, or on the next day, by the appearance of irregular groups of small, round, deep-seated, flat-topped vesicles, containing clear serum, having no inflammatory areola around them, and resembling boiled sago grains. These vesicles usually dry up in a few days, and are followed by slight desquamation; in some more severe cases, however, they enlarge, and by their confluence produce bullæ, which vary in size from a pin's head

N

to $\frac{1}{4}$ or $\frac{1}{3}$ of an inch in diameter, and are scattered over the whole palm or sole. They also dry up in a few days, and the cuticle subsequently desquamates, but occasionally the bullæ burst and then desiccate, leaving red dry patches like psoriasis. The serum, at first clear, may become, if the bullæ last a few days, opalescent and slightly yellowish, but never purulent, and it always remains alkaline.

Frequently the nails are undermined and broken near the root.

Diagnosis.—The rapid and symmetrical development, the short course and tendency to spontaneous cure, the liability to recur, and its occurrence in those of nervous temperament and the worried and over-worked, suffice to distinguish it from eczema.

The spontaneous cure and the absence of burrows separate it from scabies.

It differs from sudamina in the fluid being alkaline—not, as in sweat, acid from the beginning—a fact which is against the theory of the dependence of the disease on obstruction of the sweat ducts.

Prognosis.—The disease runs a favourable course in a few days, and is only troublesome through the itching and burning sensation it excites and from its unsightly appearance.

Treatment.—The application of lotio carbonis detergens ($\mathfrak{Z}$ ij to $\mathfrak{Z}$ vj), of vaseline, or of vaseline and liquor plumbi ($\mathfrak{m}$ xxx to $\mathfrak{Z}$ j), will usually relieve the itching. To combat the general nervous symptoms tonics may be given, of which iron, quinine, and nux vomica are the best, combined with change of air and rest.

PRURITUS.

Definition.—Pruritus is a functional disorder of the skin, arising either spontaneously or as a symptom in the course of various diseases, attended with intense itching. The scratching which it induces may cause excoriations, eczematous or pustular eruptions, and other secondary changes in the skin.

Symptoms.—Pruritus itself is usually merely a symptom produced by—

1. Local irritants, pediculi, acari, ascarides in the rectum, &c.

2. Constitutional conditions, such as jaundice, diabetes, intestinal, uterine, and genito-urinary disorders, senile decay of the skin, rheumatism, gout, &c.

The chief varieties described are—

a. Pruritus senilis, occurring in old people in association with atrophic changes in the skin. The itching, often intense, induces scratching, from which papules, excoriations, pustules, &c., result. It may be excited by pediculi corporis, in which case the marks of scratching are most distinct on the neck and shoulders.

b. Pruritus ani is a frequent and distressing accompaniment of piles, gout, uterine and other disorders.

c. Pruritus genitalium is most frequent in women, and is usually a symptom of local disease, eczema, &c., of utero-ovarian irritation, or of general diseases, such as diabetes and gout.

Diagnosis.—The intense itching, unattended by special morbid changes beyond those that are the result of scratching, suffices to distinguish it from other diseases of the skin.

Prognosis.—Pruritus, though not fatal, is often obstinate and causes great distress.

Morbid Anatomy.—No special changes have been found in the skin or cutaneous nerves.

Treatment.—The indications are—

1. To remove or mitigate any local irritation exciting the affection, and to treat constitutional symptoms or diseases of adjacent organs.

2. When no obvious cause can be found, to give tonics, iron, quinine, cod-liver oil, and locally to apply sedative lotions, such as lotio calaminæ, lotio boracis with hydrocyanic acid or dilute carbonis detergens.

N 2

When the itching is general, alkaline baths often give great relief, after which an ointment of chloral camphor ʒss to vaseline ʒj may be used with advantage. Scratching must be strictly forbidden.

DYSTROPHIA CUTIS.

Definition.—Certain changes in the skin, other than zoster, usually of an atrophic, inflammatory, or gangrenous nature, which arise under the direct influence of lesions of the nervous system.

Symptoms.—The appearances met with may be arranged under the heads—

1. Atrophic or ' glossy skin.'
2. Œdematous.
3. Eruptive, erythematous, papular, vesicular, or bullous.
4. Ulcerative and gangrenous, ' acute bed-sore.'

1. *'Glossy Skin'* is the term applied by Paget and Weir Mitchell to a peculiar condition, somewhat resembling scleroderma, which supervenes after irritative lesions of the peripheral nerves. It sometimes follows a clean cut, entirely dividing the nerve ; but more commonly a partial division, contusion, laceration, or compression in a cicatrix, callus, &c., is the cause. The skin is smooth, pale, and anæmic, or pinkish and blotched as if by chilblains, glossy, and its natural wrinkles effaced. The epidermis is often fissured, the nails are cracked and distorted, the hair is shed, and the sweat glands are atrophied, and their secretion diminished. The affected part is usually extremely tender and the seat of neuralgic pain, and its temperature is often lowered.

2. *Œdematous.*—There is often slight œdema of the skin and subcutaneous parts in paralysed limbs, which lasts for a considerable time, and gradually disappears as recovery takes place. Peculiar pale or slightly erythematous localised swellings of the skin and subcutaneous tissue, resembling chilblains, are also met with, appearing after neuralgic attacks at the sites of pain,

They are sometimes described as urticarial, but are attended by intense shooting or burning pain and not by itching.

3. *Eruptive.*—The ' lightning pains ' of locomotor ataxy, and the neuralgic attacks met with in pachymeningitis, caries, or cancer of the vertebræ, and other affections in which there is compression and irritation of the posterior nerve-roots, are often accompanied by an eruption on the painful points of skin, erythematous, papular, vesicular, pustular, or bullous in character. The patches correspond in situation, as in zoster, with the distribution of cutaneous nerves, and in their course and duration resemble that disease.

4. *Ulcerative and gangrenous* patches may occur as the sequelæ of the last-mentioned changes, or as an independent form in the ' acute bed-sore,' to which special attention has been directed by Charcot. This lesion, of grave and usually fatal import in the prognosis of cerebral or spinal diseases, appears, according to this authority, a few days, or occasionally only some hours, after the onset of the nerve symptoms, as an erythematous patch of variable extent and irregular shape, seated, in spinal disease, over the sacrum, in cerebral usually on one of the buttocks. The colour, at first light red or somewhat bluish, fades on pressure, and in some spinal cases there is a phlegmonous-looking infiltration, attended sometimes with anæsthesia, at other times with severe pain. After a day or two vesicles or bullæ, containing clear brownish or sanguineous fluid, appear in the centre of the patch; these soon burst, exposing a bright red base, dotted with purplish-black spots of cutaneous hæmorrhage, which often extends as deep as the sub-cutaneous tissue or muscles. The purple spots soon become confluent, necrose, and form a black slough surrounded by a margin of erythema. Patients rarely live long enough for the slough to be cast off, but in more chronic cases septicæmia and gangrenous meningitis soon prove fatal. These patches appear even when the most scrupulous care is taken to avoid pressure or any irritation of the skin from the urine or fæces.

Diagnosis.—The occurrence of these phenomena in connection with severe diseases of the nervous system, their restriction to certain special sites, usually related to the cutaneous distribution of nerves, and the presence, before or throughout their course, of neuralgic pain, will clearly indicate their nature.

Prognosis.—As these skin manifestations are merely symptomatic, their prognosis is that of the diseases in which they occur.

' Acute bed-sore' is, according to Charcot, an omen of a fatal result.

Morbid Anatomy.—The cutaneous appearances in the erythematous, vesicular, and other eruptions are the same as those in the simple diseases. In 'acute bed-sore' there is an exudation into the whole corium, with leucocytes and plasma, resembling phlegmonous erysipelas, which is followed later on by hæmorrhagic infiltration and gangrene.

Treatment.—This falls beyond the scope of this work. In 'acute bed-sore' keeping the part clean, the frequent application of some antiseptic lotion or powder to diminish the risk of septicæmia, and poultices to promote the separation of the sloughs should be employed.

183

CHAPTER XVII.

Class IV.—HYPERTROPHIÆ.

Ephelis — Lentigo — Melanoderma — Morbus Addisonii — Chloasma uterinum — Ichthyosis — Xeroderma — Morphœa — Scleroderma — Sclerema neonatorum — Elephantiasis Arabum — Elephantiasis teleangiectodes—Dermatolysis.

Pigmentary.

1. Ephelis and Lentigo.　2. Melanoderma.　3. Morbus Addisonii.
4. Chloasma uterinum.

EPHELIS AND LENTIGO—FRECKLES.

FRECKLES are light or dark brown spots, varying in size from a pin's head to a lentil, occurring on the skin of fair or red-haired people. They are found usually on the more exposed regions of the body, such as the face, neck, and backs of the hands and wrists, but appear also on other parts. They are greatly influenced by light, and are always darker in summer than in winter. Some doubt exists whether they can be produced by the sun's rays, but there is reason to believe that many spots otherwise imperceptible are only then visible. Exposure of the limbs to heat will often produce a similar discoloration as the result of a deposit of pigment in the rete. The appearance of the spots is entirely unattended by itching, or indeed any local or constitutional symptom. When the stains are larger, more persistent, and are not influenced by exposure to heat and cold, they are termed *lentigines.*

MELANODERMA.

This term includes all cases in which dark stains are produced through some special condition of the body, such as pregnancy, intemperance, &c.

MORBUS ADDISONII.

In the course of this disease, which is an affection of the suprarenal capsules, a remarkable bronzing of the skin takes place. After the disease has been progressing for some time, the skin is noticed to be of a darker tint than normal, a change often attributed to jaundice. The upper part of the body is usually affected earlier than the lower, but the entire surface becomes eventually involved, the colour becoming gradually darker, and—although the shades of colour vary in different cases from a light to a dark brown—in the majority of fatal cases the colour deepens markedly as death approaches. In parts where pigment is usually deposited, such as the axillæ, flexor surfaces of joints, genitals, nipples, freckles, &c., the shades will be found to be of a darker brown, or even black, making the rest of the skin appear white by contrast.

CHLOASMA UTERINUM.

This term is applied to the pigmentary deposits occurring in women suffering from uterine disease, or as a result of pregnancy. It usually appears in the form of crescentic patches on the forehead and below the hair.

Epidermis and Papillæ.

ICHTHYOSIS AND XERODERMA.

Definition.—Ichthyosis is a congenital hypertrophic disease of the skin, characterised by increased growth of the papillary layer with thickening of the true skin and the production of masses of epidermic scales.

Symptoms.—Some doubt exists whether ichthyosis is always a congenital disease. The characteristic appearance of the skin is sometimes not developed until some years after birth ; it is, however, impossible to say that some abnormal condition or tendency did not exist at birth, although it may not have become apparent until a later period, and this view is supported by the fact that ichthyosis is hereditary.

There are many degrees of ichthyosis, ranging from a mere roughness of the skin to a condition resembling that of the skin of the shark. In a case of average severity the growth of the papillary layer is greatly increased, and the whole skin thickened. The natural furrows of the skin are, as the result of this growth, much deepened, and the surface is mapped out into polygonal tracts, presenting an appearance similar to a crocodile's hide. Surmounting the ridges are collections of epidermic scales, which at first are limited in quantity, but as time progresses increase in size. Masses are formed in the centre of a patch, either thin and pearl-coloured or of varying shades of colour, from green to brown or black, and may also cover the enlarged papillæ, forming projections from the surface. There is a complete absence of perspiration from the parts attacked with the disease, but the unaffected regions, such as the head, usually perspire freely.

Ichthyosis simplex, or *Xeroderma,* is the form most frequently met with. It usually becomes apparent in the child at about two years of age, when it is nothing more than a general roughness of the skin, especially marked over the knees and elbows. At a later period the epidermis is shed in flakes and the general roughness is greatly increased, but certain regions, such as the inside of the extremities and the palms and soles, differ from healthy skin only slightly, while the face is dry and furfuraceous. With the exception of these regions the skin is covered with the irregular-shaped patches above described, limited by the natural folds of the skin. On the knees and elbows, on the fronts of the ankles and margins of the axillæ, and, indeed, on all parts exposed to friction, the masses become so thick and black from dirt that the disease is far more marked than on the other regions.

Ichthyosis cornea occurs less frequently than the simple variety. It consists of a growth of hard, horny prominences, often standing out a quarter of an inch, which, being aggregated together, form patches somewhat resembling the condition found on the knees and elbows in ichthyosis simplex. They are believed to be due to an alteration of the lining of the sebaceous follicles into horny material. This first distends the follicle, and then passes through its orifice to the surface, where it protrudes. The exposed end is broken away, and with it a part of the material in the follicle, and a cup is thus left, which is again filled by further growth of the horny substance. When these are thrown off the skin of the part is left in a normal condition.

Diagnosis.—With the exception of psoriasis there is no disease for which ichthyosis could be mistaken.

For diagnosis from psoriasis see Chapter XIII., p. 150.

Prognosis.—Ichthyosis is a very intractable disease, but is never fatal. It can be somewhat benefited by remedies, but only temporarily. Occasionally, after a prolonged and severe general illness, the disease has been observed to disappear, and has not again returned.

Morbid Anatomy.—Vertical sections show a dense accumulation of horny epidermic cells, containing frequently a considerable quantity of fatty matter ; the rete cells, especially between the papillæ, are more numerous and sometimes pigmented ; and the papillæ themselves are greatly enlarged and elongated, and contain dilated vessels and numerous cells. In severe cases the hair follicles are more or less atrophied, the sweat and sebaceous glands are wasted, and there is induration and sclerosis of the corium and atrophy of the adipose tissue.

Treatment.—Any local application likely to soften and remove the accumulated epidermis is the proper treatment, and for this purpose alkaline lotions, and soaps of various kinds, the one recommended by Hebra being composed of iodide of sulphur, oil, glycerine, have been tried. Absolute cleanliness is most

essential, and the constant and prolonged soaking of the body
in water will often lead to a diminution of the ichthyotic
condition. Various internal remedies have been tried, but with
no benefit.

Connective Tissue.

1. Morphœa.   2. Scleroderma.   3. Sclerema neonatorum.   4. Elephantiasis Arabum.   5. Elephantiasis teleangiectodes.   6. Dermatolysis.

MORPHŒA—ADDISON'S KELOID.

Definition.—Morphœa is a rare chronic affection of the skin,
characterised by the occurrence—most often on the face—of
roundish or oval, pale pink or ivory-coloured patches, which
are firm and inelastic, and therefore are not easily pinched up
into folds.

Symptoms.—Patches of 1 to 3 inches in diameter appear on
the skin in the course of some cutaneous nerve, with a pale
yellowish or ivorylike centre, smooth surface, and a well-defined
violet or lilac-tinted margin. The corium, apparently dense
and thickened, appears to be bound down to the subcutaneous
tissue. A feeling of burning or tingling sometimes attends the
development of the patches, and there may be slight pain on
pressure, but usually no alteration in cutaneous sensibility.

When the patches appear on the face they are sharply
limited by the middle line, and may occur in the area of distribution of the supra-orbital nerve or other branches of the fifth,
but on the trunk and limbs they are arranged in a somewhat
similar manner as in herpes. Pigment is occasionally deposited
in the skin around the patch, and its absence or presence
distinguishes the varieties morphœa alba and morphœa nigra.
Owing to the infiltration and rigidity of the skin, the movements
of the facial muscles and of the joints, when the skin of these
parts is the seat of the disease, are much impaired, so that the
fingers remain semiflexed and cannot be either bent or extended,
and the expression of the face becomes stony and fixed, like that

of a frozen corpse. The sweat and sebaceous secretions and the growth of hair on the hide-bound patches are frequently deficient, and the temperature is usually 2° to 3° Fahr. lower than that of the healthy skin, but there is no special trophic change in the parts affected.

The morphœa patches slowly extend, and having reached their acme may in the course of years gradually fade and leave the skin perfectly normal or only slightly pigmented. However, occasionally sclerosis takes place, and the thin, rigid skin acquires a shrunken, parchmentlike appearance, which has been termed morphœa atrophica.

Diagnosis.—Patches of morphœa differ from leucoderma, which they resemble in colour and definition, by the hard, infiltrated, and inelastic consistence of the affected skin.

The pale patches of lepra maculosa differ from those of morphœa by being anæsthetic in their centre and usually symmetrical in their distribution, while the former disease is accompanied by affections of the nerves, cutaneous tubercles, &c., which never occur in morphœa.

Keloid can hardly be mistaken for morphœa, so forcible is the contrast between the raised, pinkish, clawlike nodule of the former and the level, pale, smooth patches of the latter.

Prognosis.—Morphœa is never fatal. The disease in some cases tends slowly towards involution, and the normal elastic condition of the skin is restored; but when sclerosis and atrophy have occurred, permanent deformity is the result.

Morbid Anatomy.—See SCLERODERMA.

Treatment.—No local treatment has proved of any avail, but as general remedies tonics, such as iron, quinine, and cod-liver oil, are indicated if the case is complicated by anæmia or struma.

SCLERODERMA—SCLERIASIS.

Definition.—A rare disease of the skin, in which diffuse infiltrated and rigid areæ are met with over comparatively large portions of the surface of the body.

Symptoms.—Scleroderma begins most frequently on the back of the neck or upper extremities as a slightly raised brownish-red or pale waxy-coloured patch, and may spread more or less rapidly over the face, arm, or even over the whole body, or it may take the form of long ribbonlike streaks or patches scattered over the body and limbs. As in morphœa, the skin is thickened, inelastic, and adherent to the deeper tissues, so that it cannot be pinched up, and feels both colder and dryer than the normal skin. Irregular spots of pigment are sometimes met with on or round the patches. Sensibility is sometimes slightly impaired, and the temperature of the part is diminished 1° or 2° Fahr. The epidermis is normal, but may desquamate, and vesicles or other eruptions can appear upon it as on healthy skin. The secretions of the sweat and sebaceous glands are usually, but not invariably, diminished.

When scleroderma is first developed there is a slight localised raised swelling, produced by œdema in the subcutaneous tissue, pitting on pressure and gradually becoming sclerosed. But as the disease progresses the patches become level with or slightly depressed below the surface of the adjacent skin, and in the variety characterised by the presence of long bands the healthy skin rises on each side of them. The indurated patches subsequently, like those of morphœa, either undergo complete resolution or sclerosis and atrophy. The mucous membrane of the mouth, the tongue, and the pharynx sometimes presents similar hard white patches. Patches of morphœa may precede or accompany the development of scleroderma, and the edge of a sclerodermatous patch not unfrequently presents an appearance identical with morphœa. The differences in form and colour are comparatively unimportant in view of the resemblances in the rigid, infiltrated condition of the skin, the similarity, if not identity, of the anatomical changes, the chronic course ending in atrophy or resolution of the affected portions of skin, and the retention of the cutaneous sensibility observed in both affections. Hence morphœa and scleroderma, if not merely stages of the same disease, are certainly due to variations in the intensity and exact localisation of the same morbid process, and bear the same relation to one another as lupus erythematosus does to lupus vulgaris. In morphœa the unsymmetrical character of the patches, their abrupt limitation by the middle line, their arrangement along the course of cutaneous nerves, as in zoster, in lines or clusters, the occasional check to the development of the bones of a limb, and the slow course, unaffected by treatment, are points which strongly support the theory advocated by Mr. Hutchinson, that, like zoster, the primary cause of the disease is an affection of the nervous system.

When scleroderma attacks the face, the countenance becomes fixed, the normal folds of the skin disappear, the lips and eyelids are rigid and sometimes everted, and the movements of the jaws and neck are interfered with, owing to the want of elasticity of the skin.

In the extremities the firm, tendinous bands stiffen the joints, which then become semiflexed and almost immovable, and sometimes deep-seated pains are left in the fasciæ and bones. When atrophy of the skin has set in the subcutaneous tissue and muscles waste away, the thin, shrivelled, smooth, and reddish band of pigmented cutis appears to be in direct contact with the bones, and the wasted limb has a dried-up, skeleton-like appearance, which is persistent.

Diagnosis.—Morphœa differs from scleroderma in the form of its patches, which are round or oval and usually small, instead of being ribbonlike and covering a large area, and in their colour, which is violet or lilac-coloured at its sharply defined margin, surrounded usually by a deeply pigmented ring, and yellowish in its central portion as compared with the pale white of scleroderma.

Prognosis.—Like morphœa, scleroderma never causes death, though helplessness and great deformity may result from it. The patches occasionally undergo spontaneous resolution, and the skin resumes its normal character.

Morbid Anatomy.—Sections of the skin in this disease show a general thickening and induration of the corium, which passes gradually into and is fused with the subcutaneous fatty tissue. Microscopically examined, the epidermis is found to be normal, excepting that the rete cells contain some granular pigment. The papillæ are unchanged in shape, but their connective-tissue stroma is much more condensed, and forms a narrow meshwork of condensed fibrous bundles. The connective-tissue fibres of the corium are much thickened, form a compressed feltwork, and invade the subdermic fatty tissue, broad, dense bundles replacing the thin fibrils between groups of fat cells and compressing them firmly. Cords and networks of round and spindle cells are also found surrounding the fat cells. The vessels in many places are narrowed and surrounded by round and spindle cells, but are not usually obliterated or deficient in number. Sebaceous and sweat glands and hair follicles are but little, if at all, altered, and the arrectores pilorum are distinct. In extreme cases the sclerotic changes extend throughout the subcutaneous tissue, which is much atrophied, even down to the fascia of the muscles, and there is considerable increase in number of the elastic fibres.

The disease is considered to begin in the cellular deposits round the vessels, and in the stage of infiltration to spread thence in cords along the connective-tissue bundles. As the cellular infiltration becomes converted into fibrous and elastic tissue the sclerosis of the skin observed in the latter stages is gradually developed.

The anatomical changes in morphœa have not yet been completely investigated, but are probably analogous to those in scleroderma.

Treatment.—No specific internal remedy or local treatment has any effect on the disease, but nutritious diet, good hygiene, and tonics are recommended.

SCLEREMA NEONATORUM.

Definition.—An acute œdema and induration of the skin, occurring in young children.

Symptoms.—The cause of this disease is not well understood, but it is believed to be due to some alteration in the condition of the capillaries, resulting from some previously existing disease, such as affections of the intestines, lung, or brain, or some congenital defect. It may also result from impaired nutrition or syphilis.

It commences with swelling of the lower extremities, following œdema and induration of the skin of the part, which is itself tense, shining, pits on pressure, and of a red, white, or livid colour.

After a time, varying from a few hours to two or three days, the swelling subsides, leaving the skin wrinkled; sometimes, however, the advanced stage of wrinkling of the skin is the first symptom, and is not preceded by the earlier stage of œdema. The general condition of the child is much altered, and it shows but few signs of vitality, while the temperature is lowered by two or three degrees. The disease gradually spreads upwards till the skin of the face is affected, when the features become immovable and neither the eyes nor mouth can be opened. The reduction of temperature and the loss of vitality continue till death results after from two to ten days' illness.

Diagnosis.—This disease resembles no other. A local œdema cannot be mistaken for it for more than a few hours, and the general condition then suffices to distinguish between the two.

Prognosis.—It is usually fatal.

Morbid Anatomy.—Few changes have been found beyond a more or less œdematous infiltration of the whole skin and a rigid condition of the subcutaneous connective tissue. A slight increase of connective tissue in the deeper corium layer, and nodules and cords of embryonic tissue in the panniculus adiposus between the fat cells, have also been described by some authors.

Treatment.—This consists in first removing the primary cause, when it can be ascertained, and afterwards in restoring, when possible, the circulation through the capillaries of the affected part.

ELEPHANTIASIS ARABUM.

Definition.—Elephantiasis Arabum is an enlargement of some part of the body, usually a limb, due to hypertrophy of the whole of the connective tissue, following an inflammatory condition of the part.

Symptoms.—Under the name of elephantiasis several entirely distinct diseases have been included, and much confusion has resulted from the indiscriminate use of the word ; thus, elephantiasis Græcorum is simply leprosy, and elephantiasis Italica is another name for pellagra. It is especially common in hot climates, such as the west coast of Africa, Barbadoes, and Malabar. Its prevalence is not confined to any particular sex, age, or race, but various conditions have been suspected to be concerned in its etiology. It has been attributed to injuries of the veins and lymphatics, which have caused compression, and to lupus, and apparently with some reason to the gummata of syphilis. Elephantiasis Arabum begins with an erysipelatous inflammation of the skin, usually of the leg, which is accompanied with or preceded by feverishness and symptoms of general constitutional disturbance resembling intermittent fever. These symptoms gradually subside, but some amount of swelling of the skin remains. After a variable interval the inflammation of the skin, with redness, swelling, and pain returns again, accompanied with or preceded by symptoms of constitutional disturbance. The same subsidence takes place, but the local effects last longer than in the previous attack, and leave a greater amount of permanent œdematous swelling behind them. These attacks are repeated from time to time during a series of years, and thus a gradual enlargement of the limb takes place until it has attained huge proportions.

The skin is greatly thickened, shiny, stretched, and of a colour varying from light brown to purple. Desquamation may be present, or the skin may be smooth and frequently fissured, when the natural furrows are greatly exaggerated,

o

owing to the thickening of the skin, and when the epidermis is heaped up and macerated by perspiration. The surface may be surmounted with tubercles, the result of growth of fibro-cellular tissue, or with large papillæ, which may or may not be covered with epidermis. Sometimes the whole limb is covered with eczema, and occasionally the skin ulcerates, forming sores of varying size, from which a foul discharge exudes. Enlargement of the lymphatics causes them to stand up on the surface like vesicles, and when they burst or are punctured the milky lymph escapes. Each attack is accompanied by stabbing pains in the limb, but they are more severe at the beginning than at any subsequent period. Severe pain is, however, always felt if the limb be allowed to be in a dependent position for any length of time. Diminution of the sensibility of the surface also results from the disease. The enormous increase of the leg and foot when that part is affected causes the obliteration of the instep and upper part of the foot, and makes it resemble the foot of an elephant, whence the peculiar name.

Elephantiasis of the genitals differs slightly from that of any other part, and affects the scrotum, penis, labia, and clitoris. It commences 'in the form of a hard kernel under the skin, usually at the bottom of the left side of the scrotum.' From this point the disease spreads, and the skin over it becomes thickened and wrinkled, while the shape of the abdomen undergoes alteration. The penis is also increased in size, but lies partially embedded in the enlarged scrotum. The skin of its lower surface is pushed forwards, and is only connected with the penis round the glans. The hypertrophied scrotum becomes covered with dilated lymphatics, which at a later stage burst and permit lymph to exude.

The regions usually affected are the lower extremities and the genitals, but the upper extremities and ears may also be the seats of the disease.

Diagnosis.—Simple œdema is the only condition which bears the slightest resemblance to elephantiasis, but never leads to hypertrophy of the tissues.

Prognosis.—Elephantiasis may last a lifetime, and although it has no tendency to spontaneous recovery, it is, within limits, amenable to treatment.

· *Morbid Anatomy.*—Sections of a limb affected with elephantiasis show the corium thickened and much indurated, the subcutaneous connective tissue greatly increased, in some parts dense and glistening, in others soft and gelatinous ; the muscles wasted, soft, and yellowish ; the fasciæ, intermuscular tissue, and periosteum much thickened ; and the bones hypertrophied, increased in both length and thickness, and presenting frequently irregular exostoses, which sometimes unite together adjacent bones. Caries and necrosis may also be present. A clear, yellowish, coagulable lymph exudes freely from the cut surface. The veins are dilated, and in places plugged by clots, and here and there may be observed irregular spaces filled with clear lymph.

Microscopically examined, the epidermis and papillary layer are seen to be raised into rugose, prominent masses, resembling ichthyosis. In these masses the epidermic horny layers are much thickened, the rete cells pigmented, and the papillæ greatly increased in size. The corium bundles of connective tissue are increased in thickness, present a swollen, gelatinous, and glistening appearance, and are closely felted together. Fusiform and stellate cells are seen between them in places. The subcutaneous connective tissue is occasionally more than an inch thick, in some places dense and fibrous, and fused with the corium, in others soft and gelatinous, consisting of loose areolar and embryonic connective tissue, pervaded with lymph, and in the latter case it merges into the fasciæ and areolæ, which themselves present similar changes. The muscles, from atrophy and fatty degeneration, become pale, and often seem to lose their true striated fibres, which are apparently replaced by fatty and granular débris, while the nerves are also compressed, indurated, and atrophied. The blood vessels present their normal arrangement, except that they are more widely separated, owing to the increase of connective tissue. The veins, dilated and thickened in places, are sometimes thrombosed, and in later stages are indicated only by pigmented fibrous cords. The lymphatics are in places much dilated and form small cysts, the walls of which, though usually thickened, are sometimes thin and friable. The interstitial lymph spaces and canaliculi are also enlarged, and here and there form cysts filled with clear yellow lymph or gelatinous embryonic connective tissue.

When the lymphatics are ruptured they discharge abundantly, and the discharge, which consists of lymph or chylous fluid, has been found in some cases to contain filaria sanguinis hominis. The dilatations are ascribed by some authors to the irritation excited by these parasites and the obstruction caused by them in the lymph channels.

The hair follicles, sweat and sebaceous glands, much elongated and widely separated, but otherwise little altered, in the early stages of the disease, become later compressed and atrophied.

Treatment.—The first thing to be done is to allay the inflammation by complete rest and, if possible, the elevation of the part affected, and by the application of warm poultices. After the inflammation has been reduced Hebra recommends the use of baths, poultices, and ointments to remove the accumulation of epidermis, and subsequently inunction with blue ointment. Bandages must next be applied to reduce the size of the limb, and Martin's elastic bandage is probably the best for the purpose. Ligature of the main vessel of the limb has been recommended, but with such slight success as hardly to warrant its general adoption.

ELEPHANTIASIS TELEANGIECTODES.

Definition.—This disease is closely related to elephantiasis Arabum, but differs from it in that it may arise without any previous inflammation and is usually congenital.

Symptoms.—This disease is either congenital or appears soon after birth, and is due to some obstruction of the lymphatics. The skin of a limb becomes hypertrophied, and hangs down in rolls or flaps, which vary in colour, owing to the enlargement of the vessels, but if pressure be steadily exerted on one of these flaps its size becomes considerably reduced. Although the thickening of the skin which hangs from the lower part of a limb produces an apparent increase in the size of the limb, the upper part has really wasted, and this atrophy is not confined to the skin, but includes the muscles and bones. After a time a quantity of vesicles appear, which may be arranged in groups or lines or may be scattered irregularly, and when these are ruptured the lymph which they contain exudes.

Morbid Anatomy.—In elephantiasis teleangiectodes the essential morbid process is a new formation of connective tissue, at first embryonic, but later on dense and fibrous, in the subcutaneous tissue. The growths next present changes in the skin and subcutaneous tissue analogous to those in elephantiasis Arabum; they are, however, pervaded by slits, gaps, and cysts filled with lymph, and by numerous blood vessels, which are dilated, communicate freely, and sometimes become cavernous.

Treatment.—Is identical with that suggested for elephantiasis Arabum.

DERMATOLYSIS.

Definition.—Dermatolysis is a growth of the skin, causing it to hang in folds.

Symptoms.—The disease may occur in any part of the body, but according to Alibert it most frequently attacks the eyebrows, face, neck, abdomen, and labia, and is due to a pathological change in the skin, causing an increase of the fibro-cellular tissue. The skin hangs in folds, but no other symptom is present beyond some loss of sensibility in the part.

CHAPTER XVIII.

Class V.—ATROPHIÆ.'

Albinismus – Leucoderma—Atrophia cutis.

Pigmentary.

1. Albinismus. 2. Leucoderma.

ALBINISMUS.

Definition.—Albinismus is a congenital absence of pigment from the skin, hair, iris, and choroid, which may be either general or local.

Persons suffering from general deficiency or absence of pigment are termed albinos.

Symptoms.—In albinos the skin is dull white and of delicate texture, the hair is fine and yellowish or white, the iris is pink, and the choroid being devoid of the normal dark pigment, the pupil appears red instead of black. Persons thus affected are stated to be usually of delicate health, and their skins are more prone to suffer from exposure to heat and cold.

The affection is more frequently met with in the tropics, and is more noticed in the dark races.

In the partial form of the disease patches resembling leucoderma are found scattered about the body, giving the person, if dark, a piebald appearance.

Morbid Anatomy.—Microscopic examination of the skin of albinos shows absence of the normal pigment from the deeper rete cells.

Treatment.—No treatment is of any avail.

LEUCODERMA—WHITE LEPROSY.

Definition.—A local deficiency or absence of pigment from the skin and hair, developed after birth and slowly spreading, but causing no constitutional disturbance.

Symptoms.—Leucoderma begins by the appearance of one or more round white patches on various parts of the body, generally near brown moles or warts. The patch has a defined margin, bordered by a ring of excessive pigmentation, which gradually merges in the healthy skin, and the hair on the patch is also white, but the affected skin in every respect except the absence of pigment presents no structural or functional difference from healthy skin. As the patches gradually enlarge they become oval, and by confluence form large pale tracts with convex margins bounded by deeply pigmented rings. As time goes on and the white patches spread, more and more of the skin is affected, till finally only a few brown patches with concave edges are left to represent the normal skin. The disease may originate at any age, but most frequently after puberty, and is almost always bilateral, though exact symmetry is rarely found.

Diagnosis.—The pale patches of lepra maculosa or lepra anæsthetica may be distinguished from those of leucoderma in that their edges are more shaded, the skin often infiltrated and anæsthetic in the centre as well as scarred, and that they often have a purplish raised hyperæsthetic border, whereas those of leucoderma have a sharply defined border and a dark pigmented ring. The structure and functions of the skin also in the latter are normal.

The concave edges of the dark patches which represent normal skin will enable extensive leucoderma to be distinguished from abnormal development of pigment in a healthy skin.

Prognosis.—Leucoderma causes no pain or inconvenience to the person affected, but the white patches, though they some-

times become stationary, have no tendency to disappear spontaneously or under treatment.

Morbid Anatomy.—The only change that has been detected
is an absence of pigment from the deeper layers of the rete and
from the hairs and their bulbs.

Treatment.—No remedies have yet been found to remove
the white patches.

Of Connective Tissue.

ATROPHIA CUTIS.

Atrophy of the skin, besides occurring as a result of various
inflammatory affections or new growths of the skin, is met with
as an independent disease, both in a general and a partial
form.

The first condition is usually a result of retrogressive or
degenerative changes in old persons, and has been called *senile
atrophy.*

In it the skin becomes dry, wrinkled, rough, less supple,
and more or less pigmented. The epidermis is smooth, or in
places branny, the cutis and its papillæ are thinned and wasted,
and the subcutaneous fatty tissue is usually atrophied. Hairs
are scanty or wanting, and the sebaceous glands either atrophied
or presenting degeneration in the form of milium granules.
Anatomically the tissues may be found either in a condition
which is mainly that of *simple atrophy,* or, in addition, more or
less marked *degenerative metamorphoses* are present.

In the former condition of simple atrophy the cuticle is thin
and the papillæ either wanting or projecting very slightly above
the level of the corium. The corium meshes are thin, narrow,
and contain few small corpuscles and very little interstitial fluid,
while granular pigment, diffuse or in masses, is abundant. The
fat cells are wasted, and contain vacuoles in places instead of oil
globules. The vessels are thin, atrophied, and pigmented in
some places, but varicose in others, and the hair follicles, though

present, have their papillæ wasted and contain no hairs, or only their lanuginous filaments.

In the degenerative conditions, in addition to the simple atrophy, the skin, in tracts of varying extent, becomes brittle and extremely thin, while its connective-tissue bundles become converted into a vitreous or gelatinous mass, in which no vessels or nerves are visible. The hair and glandular follicles are also degenerated. The process is supposed to begin in the arterioles, like albuminoid degeneration, and to spread thence to the other tissue.

Partial atrophy of the skin is observed in the form of white, scarlike parallel bands, a half to two lines broad and several inches long, or in scattered round maculæ, a quarter to two lines in diameter.

The striæ (*linear atrophy*) which are the most common have a glistening bluish-white appearance, and the skin forming them is unduly thin and depressed. They usually occur on the pelvic brim, the glutei, and the trochanters, and less frequently on the fronts of the thighs or the arms. Under the microscope the papillary layer is found atrophied, the corium much thinned, with its bundles delicate and its vessels fewer in number, and the subcutaneous fatty tissue and appendages are wasted.

The maculæ are much less frequently observed, but Dr. Liveing has found the following changes to occur in them :— The spots, at first somewhat reddish, raised above the skin, hard and fibrous, passed on into the ordinary atrophic condition, appearing as discrete round or oval, pitlike scars, covered by a thin membrane, and all about the size of a threepenny-piece. Finally a stage of contraction or obliteration sets in, and the spots become less apparent, as if encroached upon by the surrounding healthy tissues. Liveing believes this disease to be allied to scleroderma and morphœa, with which it has been several times associated.

CHAPTER XIX.

Class VI.—NEOPLASMATA.

Sub-class A.—*Benign.*

Clavus — Tylosis — Verruca — Cornu cutaneum — Keloid — Fibroma — Xanthoma—Lupus vulgaris—Lupus erythematosus—Rhinoscleroma—Nævus—Angioma—Lymphangioma.

Papillomatous.

1. Clavus and Tylosis.   2. Verruca.   3. Cornu cutaneum.

CLAVUS AND TYLOSIS.

Definition.—Tylosis, or tyloma, is merely an undue accumulation of horny epidermis, which appears usually on the extremities, on parts exposed to pressure. The thickened epidermis merges gradually on each side into the normal, and there is little or no affection of the corium.

Clavus, or 'corn,' is the name applied to an epidermic accumulation, resembling that in tylosis, in the centre of which is a conical plug, the apex being situated on, and pressing down, the corium.

Symptoms.—Tylosis causes usually little or no inconvenience, unless the accumulation be very thick and horny. Under these circumstances, when affecting the palm, it interferes much with the movements of the hand. When irritated, a vesicle may be formed, which spreads into a bulla, the fluid, on account of its long retention, becoming purulent, and thus a sub-epidermic abscess may be produced. The horny crust is loosened and cast off, leaving, after the ulcerated base heals, a perfectly normal surface.

A ' corn,' on the other hand, causes usually depression, and atrophy of the papillæ beneath its ' core,' and when pressed upon gives rise to severe pain.   It is generally produced by the pressure of a tight boot on the toes.   When seated between the toes the maceration by retained moisture prevents it from assuming the horny character of the callosity, and hence this is the distinction between hard and soft corns.

Morbid Anatomy.—Tylosis consists of an undue thickening of the epithelium.   The horny layers are increased in number and thickness, and the papillæ are somewhat enlarged and more vascular.

Sections through a corn show an epithelial accumulation and papillary hypertrophy indentical with that in tylosis.   In the centre of the patch, however, a conical epidermic plug is found, the layers of which are concave towards the free surface of the skin.   The papillæ beneath it, at first enlarged, are gradually atrophied as the growth deepens, which causes wasting of the corium and glands, till the core finally lies in a pit in the corium.

Treatment.—Occasional rubbing down of the horny mass with a file is all that is needed in tylosis.   When affecting the palm, dressing with lint soaked in liquor potassæ and covered with oiled silk, and subsequent scraping away of the softened epidermis, restores mobility to the parts.

Corns may be treated by placing a disc of felt plaister, with a hole in the centre, over them, so as to remove pressure. Dressing with liquor potassæ or with strong nitric acid will often, after a time, cause the disappearance of the affection, and in obstinate cases excision of the corn, with the papillæ from which it grows, may be necessary.

VERRUCA—WART.

Definition.—A wart is a small excrescence of the skin, or mucous membrane near the junction with the skin, consisting of a localised hypertrophy of the papillæ and the epidermis covering them.

Symptoms.—Warts may be *hard* when exposed to the air on cutaneous surfaces, or *soft* when seated on mucous membranes, kept constantly moist by secretions; they may also be simple or compound, the latter being made up of a bunch of filiform papillæ, usually pedunculate. Simple warts consist of a group of elongated papillæ, surrounded by a common epithelial envelope, the surface of which, however, usually presents fissures marking the extent of each papilla. Hard warts, on the hands, body, and head, may appear suddenly in great numbers, and grow rapidly, and as they are also liable to involution and spontaneous disappearance, various quack remedies, ' charms,' &c., have been able to acquire an easy but somewhat doubtful reputation.

Soft warts, or condylomata, are usually pointed, and are much softer and more vascular than the hard; they occur most often on the perineum, round the anus, and on the genitals, owing to the irritation of the gonorrhœal discharge, syphilis, or decomposing sweat in persons of dirty habits. They have no tendency to spontaneous involution.

Morbid Anatomy.—In the flat warts vertical sections show merely an aggregation of hypertrophied, sometimes branched, papillæ, the vessels of which are enlarged, and the epidermis covering them is much thickened. The columnar cells of the rete are specially numerous, and fill up the interpapillary spaces. In the round, prominent, or conical warts the hypertrophied, much elongated papillæ are still embedded in a mass of thickened epithelium, which envelopes them in a common sheath; but indications of the extent of each papilla are presented by numerous fine cracks, which split it up into polygonal areæ, each corresponding to a papilla and its envelope. In the filiform warts the papillæ, delicate and branched, have each a separate epidermic coat, and the little mass appears like a bundle of fine bristles.

Treatment.—Hard warts, not showing any tendency to disappear, may be snipped off with curved scissors, and some styptic or cautery may be applied to the seat of attachment if there is any bleeding. If sessile, the repeated application of glacial acetic acid, of chromic or nitric acids or liquor potassæ, will usually cause them to shrivel up.

Condylomata may also be treated by excision and styptics if few in number. If numerous, they should be removed with Paquelin's benzoline cautery.

CORNU—HORN.

Definition.—A cutaneous horn consists of a curved, conical-ridged, brownish mass, and may be considered as a wart, the epidermis over which has a columnar structure and is closely compressed like that of the nails.

Symptoms.—Horns usually occur on the head, but sometimes on the penis, and they may be several inches long and spirally twisted. Occasionally they arise within a sebaceous follicle. Their growth is attended with little or no pain.

Treatment.—Excision of the horn, with the portion of skin from which it grows, is the only effectual cure.

Of Connective Tissue.

1. Keloid.   2. Fibroma.   3. Xanthoma.

KELOID—KELOID OF ALIBERT.

Definition.—Keloid is a rare affection of the skin, consisting in the formation, spontaneously or in the seat of former scars, of a firm nodular tumour, composed of hypertrophied fibrous tissue, tender on pressure and sometimes attended with itching and tingling.

Symptoms.—There is no essential difference between the 'spontaneous' or 'true' and the so-called 'false' keloid, developed in cicatrices, and there is some doubt whether the 'true' keloid of Alibert does not really arise in small, insignificant scars, the origin of which has been forgotten. The affection named keloid by Addison is identical with, and has been described under the head of, Morphœa.

Keloid grows slowly as a rounded, oval, fusiform, or nodular patch, raised one or more lines above the surface of the skin, in which it appears embedded. Occasionally it presents the shape of a stellate or radiating, latticelike formation, and sends out processes like the claws of a crab, which gradually subside in the surrounding skin. It is firm and elastic to the touch, has a smooth surface, is white, or occasionally pinkish, shiny, and marked by ramifying vessels. The surface is never scaly, and the tumour has no tendency at any time to ulcerate or break down. Tenderness on pressure is usually present, and sometimes tingling, itching, or burning.

The growths occur as isolated patches on the sternum, mammæ, sides of the trunk, or back; they may be single, but are more frequently multiple, and sometimes are met with all over the body. The cicatricial variety may develope in scars, present in any situation, but it is said to be more common in the dark races in the scars left by flogging. It usually occurs in adults. Kaposi states that new patches arise as follows :—

'They consist, at the commencement, of brownish-red streaks of skin, with a pale red or whitish lustre, of the size of oats or barleycorns, flat or already slightly elevated, communicating a sense of resistance, and are for the most part slightly painful on pressure. In the course of many months, or of years, the linear or streaky keloid increases in one or other direction, or in every superficial dimension, and thus assumes one of the characteristic shapes mentioned above, with or without processes. At the same time it will have become somewhat thicker and more elevated.'

Keloid, once fully developed, remains, as a rule, unaltered for life ; in only a few cases has spontaneous involution, or even complete disappearance of a single patch, been observed (Alibert and Hebra).

Clinically, keloid arising in or round about a scar is indistinguishable in its course and symptoms from the spontaneous variety.

Diagnosis.—A firm, whitish or pinkish, slightly elevated tumour in the skin, sending out clawlike processes, tender on pressure, growing slowly, and manifesting no tendency to degenerative changes, can only be a keloid or a hypertrophied scar. In course and symptoms there is no valid mark of separation between the two, and microscopic examination alone will complete the diagnosis.

Prognosis.—Keloid does not affect the general health, and causes only slight inconvenience by the tenderness and occasional tingling. When removed by operation, it almost invariably recurs, and is then larger than the previous growth.

Morbid Anatomy.—Vertical sections of a 'true' keloid tumour show a mass of dense white fibrous tissue, embedded in the substance of the corium.

Under the microscope the bundles of tissue composing it are seen to run parallel to the surface of the skin and to the long axis of the tumour. The epidermis, and papillæ covering it, are normal, and the sebaceous and sweat glands, pushed aside at the margin, but not otherwise altered, may be strangulated and degenerated in the portion of corium above and below the nodule. Nuclei, spindle cells, and connective-tissue corpuscles, almost wanting in the centre, are more abundant in the periphery, especially round the vessels which seem to form centres for the formation of the growth.

In cicatricial keloid a nodule, of the same nature, is found embedded in ordinary scar tissue, which forms a sort of capsule round it, and is covered by a layer of pigmented epithelium without papillæ.

In a hypertrophied scar the pigmented rete layer of the epidermis lies on a meshwork of irregularly interlacing fibrous bundles, the papillæ being absent. Numerous round spindle and stellate cells and blood vessels—some pervious, while others are seen as fibrous, pigmented cords— are present throughout.

Treatment.—Any attempt to remove the tumour by excision, caustics, or the actual cautery should be discouraged, on account of the speedy return and enlargement of the growth. The pain, if severe, should be mitigated by subcutaneous injection of morphia, or by an aconite ointment.

FIBROMA—MOLLUSCUM FIBROSUM.

Definition.—Small sessile, pedunculate, usually multiple growths arising in the superficial layers of the corium and of somewhat gelatinous structure.

Symptoms.—The disease begins by the appearance of small, softish masses in the skin, most commonly on the chest, back, and neck, which grow slowly, and vary in size from a small shot to a large nut. From being at first sessile, as they enlarge they become more or less pedunculated, and sometimes even pendulous. They usually occur in adults, are covered with normal skin, and cause no pain or constitutional symptoms.

Diagnosis.—The little soft, usually multiple, tumours are distinguished from molluscum contagiosum by the absence of a central umbilicus, and by the fact that they consist of solid tissue, and their contents cannot therefore be pressed out.

Prognosis.—Fibroma is troublesome only on account of the deformity it causes; it is, as a rule, unattended with pain, and is in no way dangerous to life.

Morbid Anatomy.—The little growths present a whitish centre and gelatinous margin, and on microscopic examination are found to consist, in the centre, of young connective tissue, the meshes of which contain abundant serous fluid with some spindle and round cells, while the periphery may be composed of more or less mucoid tissue, with numerous branched and spindle cells. The growth, according to Rindfleisch, begins in the papillary layer.

Treatment.—The only measure of any avail is the removal of the tumours by operation, which should only be undertaken. if they cause considerable deformity or if, by pressing on nerves, they give rise to pain or inconvenience. If pendulous, a ligature

may be used, or they may be snipped off with scissors. As numerous vessels enter their base, sharp bleeding may follow their
removal by operation, but this can be usually stopped by pressure.

XANTHOMA—XANTHELASMA—VITILIGOIDEA.

Definition.—Xanthoma consists in the formation of yellow
or buff-coloured, clearly defined patches in the skin, on a level
with it or only slightly raised, and most frequently in association with prolonged jaundice.

Symptoms.—Xanthoma occurs in adults, and about twice
as frequently in women as in men. It may be localised
and limited to the eyelids only, where it usually begins, or
patches may be found scattered all over the surface of the body,
in the mucous membranes, and in the sheaths of tendons.

Two forms are described—

1. Xanthoma planum.   2. Xanthoma tuberosum.

1. *Xanthoma planum* begins, usually symmetrically, near
the inner canthus, and extends slowly along both lids, especially
the upper one, spreading thence over the adjacent part of the
cheek where the skin is thin. The patches, of different sizes,
and varying in colour from yellowish white to a faded buff or a
chamois-leather tint, have sharply defined margins, a smooth
surface level with the skin or raised into little tubercles at the
edges. There is no difference, in consistence or thickness, between the affected and the healthy skin, and usually no subjective symptoms are present.

2. *Xanthoma tuberosum* occurs as isolated nodules, or
plaques, made up of aggregations of little tubercles, varying in
size from a millet seed to a grain of wheat, just slightly raised
above the level of the skin. They occur but rarely on the eyelids, more often on the cheeks and ears, hands and feet, and
sometimes generally over the whole surface of the body. They
can be pinched up with the skin, with which they are continuous,
have a feeling of elasticity, and are attended with slight tender-

P

ness on pressure. On the palms and soles, however, they often
cause severe pricking and burning pain, which interferes much
with the use of the limb. Both forms of xanthoma not unfrequently occur in the same individual. The patches, growing
slowly by extension or by the formation of new marginal spots,
reach their full development, and remain unaltered for the rest
of life, undergoing no degenerative changes and causing no impairment of the general health. They have been observed in
various diseases, and even in healthy persons, but in a large
number of cases—in 15 out of 30 enumerated by Kaposi—persistent jaundice has preceded or accompanied them. Whether,
however, the jaundice—produced most frequently, according to
Charcot, by hypertrophic cirrhosis—is the cause of the skin
affection, or whether both phenomena are due to some other
factor, is as yet unsettled.

Diagnosis.—Xanthoma may be mistaken for confluent
masses of milium, especially on the eyelids. A superficial cut
over the mass enables the milium granules to be easily squeezed
out, whereas xanthoma, being embedded in and continuous
with the healthy corium, cannot thus be enucleated.

Prognosis.—Xanthoma is in no way dangerous to life, exerts
no influence on the general health, and is annoying only from
its unsightliness and from the pain when on the palms or soles.

Morbid Anatomy.—Vertical sections show a pale red surface, interspersed with yellow spots which cannot be squeezed
out. Under the microscope the papillæ and epidermis are
almost normal, the only change being the deposit of much yellowish pigment in the rete cells and throughout the corium.
In the cutis the yellow spots are made up of densely fibrillated
connective tissue, with more or less abundant stellate or roundish
cells intermixed. The changes are most marked round the hair
follicles and sebaceous glands. Pigment granules are scattered
throughout, but the yellow colour is due mainly to fat, which
occurs as fine globules in the stellate cells, or as a coarsely
granular mass with some large globules between and in the
connective-tissue bundles. The change differs from atheroma,

which it much resembles, in being an infiltration, and not a degeneration, of the new-formed connective tissue.

Treatment.—The excision of the whole nodule down to the subcutaneous tissue, in such a place that the scar will not subsequently cause interference with the functions of the part, is the only remedy.

Granulation-tissue Growths.

1. Lupus vulgaris. 2. Lupus erythematosus. 3. Rhinoscleroma.

LUPUS.

Definition.—A chronic, non-infectious disease, consisting in the deposit of nests of small round cells, irregularly placed in the substance of the corium, or more specially round the vessels in the plexuses of sweat and sebaceous glands. The deposits terminate either in interstitial absorption or in breaking down and ulceration, and leave superficial scars.

Symptoms.—Though various forms of lupus have been described under separate names, and the distinctions laid down are sufficiently marked in typical instances, the occurrence, in practice, of various transitional forms, and the presence, occasionally, of two varieties in the same individual, tend to show that the different varieties of lupus are due, like those of eczema, merely to local peculiarities of site, and to degrees of development of one or other of the morbid phenomena met with in the disease. Thus in lupus vulgaris the cellular new growth is well-marked, and may either be confined to the upper layer of the skin, or disseminated in nodules, or diffused through the whole thickness of the corium, while in lupus erythematosus the hyperæmia of the plexus round the sebaceous glands is the main feature, the new growth being but small.

Lupus vulgaris occurs at first as small reddish or yellowish brown nodules—presenting an 'apple-jelly' appearance—about the size of a pin's head or shot, either diffusely scattered or aggregated closely in groups in the substance of the skin.

They are not raised, and get paler, but do not disappear on pressure, and are covered by smooth epidermis. They may be quite superficial or deep in the substance of the corium, and enlarge slowly, new nodules appearing as the old reach their full development. The firm, transparent masses thus formed are painless, and often, by confluence, form flattened plaques, the size of a sixpence or larger, raised about a line above the level of the surface, irregular or smooth and covered by shiny desquamating epithelium. By continued growth of the nodules projecting tubercles may be formed, and persist without change for a long time.

As the disease progresses either involution or ulceration may take place. In the former the tubercle becomes flaccid, the skin over it shrunken and wrinkled, and covered with white scales or scabs, which on falling off leave a central white, glistening, cicatricial depression, that is firm and contracts but little. In the latter the tubercle softens, disintegrates, and secretes pus, which dries up, forming thin yellowish or greenish crusts, resting on a depressed ulcer, with soft, defined edges and a red, smooth, bleeding base. As time goes on the skin between the granulations is more or less thoroughly destroyed, the tendons, fasciæ, and other subcutaneous structures attacked, and an ulcer is formed with hard or undermined edges, and a base, covered with exuberant or friable granulations, which heals but slowly after it may be weeks, months, or even years. But while retrogression may be going on in one part, new nodules are constantly appearing in the margin of the patch, in skin previously free, or even in cicatrices left by the healing process, and thus the disease is constantly spreading. By the contact and fusion of two or more circular patches a gyrate appearance is produced, known as *lupus serpiginosus*. When the disease is superficial, and shrivels up without ulceration, it is called *lupus non-exedens*; when the growth forms prominent masses, *lupus tuberculatus*; *lupus exedens* and *lupus exulcerans* when ulceration has taken place; and *lupus exfoliaceus* when it is undergoing absorption with desquamation, and not sloughing. Lupus vulgaris arises most commonly between

the second and eighteenth years of life, and tends to disappear
with advancing age, though relapses may occur at any period.
It is rather more often met with in women than in men, is non-
contagious, and though often and certainly associated with a
strumous or phthisical diathesis, it does not appear to be hereditary. Lupus generally attacks the skin of the different parts of
the body in the following order : the cheeks, the nose, the ears, the
wrists, and the trunk. On the cheeks and nose it occurs usually
as disseminated tubercles, which, after disappearance, leave the
skin in a white, glistening, hairless condition, slightly pitted with
scars. The mucous membrane of the mouth, nares, and fauces
may be affected by extension of the disease from the nose and
cheeks, in the nose the extension of the granulation tissue inwards
to the mucous membrane eroding, and often replacing, the cartilage, and subsequently breaking down and giving rise to loss of
substance and serious deformity. On the extremities lupus is
usually serpiginous, though scattered spots may be found. The
cicatrices which it produces may keep the elbows, knees, and
fingers semiflexed and in a state of pseudo-ankylosis. In addition to this, lupus of the extremities is specially prone to
erysipelas and lymphangitis, with occasional subcutaneous
abscesses, and to the occurrence of periostitis, caries, and necrosis of the bones.

Lupus erythematosus begins usually as a reddish patch on
the nose, with slightly irregular surface, followed soon by the
development, on each cheek, of similar red patches. An erythematous spot, caused by heat or sunburn, or a small patch of
eczema, may be the starting point. On close examination the
patches appear simply erythematous, and may come and go
for some time before the disease becomes established, or they
may be made up of an aggregation of slightly raised red spots,
about the size of a pin's head, which become pale on pressure,
and often present a light greasy scale in the centre. They constitute, according to Kaposi, the 'primary eruptive spots' of
the affection, and each corresponds with the opening of a
sebaceous follicle, the little scale, made up of epidermis and

sebum, sending a small conical plug down into the duct of the gland. In severe cases, where the spots are closely aggregated, the scales become rapidly confluent, and form an irregular, closely adherent crust. When this has been softened by oil and removed, numerous little processes, passing from its under surface into the follicles, can be seen, distinguishing it in the diagnosis from acute eczema.

When the spots remain discrete, they spread gradually at the margin, which is red, slightly raised, and covered with scales and comedones, while the centre becomes pale, depressed, and pitted.

In this way the patches join at the bridge of the nose, and the characteristic ' butterfly' outline is produced, the portions on the cheeks representing the wings and that on the nose the body. Growing in this manner, the patches may spread to the scalp, or cover the whole side of the face, and new spots may develope on the ears, generally symmetrically, leaving a band of healthy skin between them and the cheek.

After persisting for a long time, often many years, the margins of the patch become paler, flatter, and gradually cease to grow, leaving a white superficial, slightly pitted scar, which may persist for the rest of life, or in process of time become almost imperceptible. Next to the cheeks, nose, and ears, the backs of the hands are most commonly affected, and it is rare for one hand only to suffer, the disease here, as elsewhere, preserving its tendency to symmetry.

In the disseminated and aggregated form (Kaposi) the individual spots do not spread at their margins as in the previously described or discoid variety, but run their course and cicatrise, leaving small pitted scars like those of acne or variola, and extension of the patches occurs by the development of new isolated spots in the adjacent tissue. Appearing first on the face, the patches may be confined to it or may spread thence to the scalp, neck, arms, and even the fingers and toes. At the onset the patch may be covered by an impetiginous scab, which, falling off after some days, exposes the primary eruptive spots.

This form of lupus erythematosus is usually chronic, but may occur acutely, either primarily or supervening on the discoid or aggregated variety. Patches of densely aggregated spots appear first on the face, and in the course of a few days are followed by the eruption of hundreds of lupus spots all over the general surface. Other local and constitutional symptoms of some severity usually accompany the outburst. Of these Kaposi enumerates the following :—

1. Subcutaneous, painful, and tender nodules, of doughy consistency, covered at first by normal skin, which in two or three days, as the swelling begins to subside, present a crop of primary eruptive spots.

2. Painful œdematous swellings of the skin and tissues round the joints of the hands and feet, and sometimes of the knee and elbow also, which, after some days, subside gradually with the development of spots of lupus erythematosus.

3. Large, hard, painful swellings of the submaxillary and axillary, and more rarely the inguinal and parotid glands, subsiding with the development of the eruption usually within a few weeks.

4. Erysipelas, or lymphangitis, only occurring chiefly in acute attacks in the parts affected by the painful subcutaneous swellings, and on the face and ears. It may also arise, in chronic cases, even if no operation have been performed, lupus erythematosus being more liable to it than lupus vulgaris. It is usually a grave complication, and is frequently fatal.

Diagnosis. Lupus vulgaris.—The presence in the skin of the characteristic 'apple-jelly' nodules is sufficient in itself for the diagnosis. Scabs, if present, should be removed by oiling, and if no spots are then discovered, waiting for a few weeks will usually enable the gradual development of new nodules to be seen.

From syphilis, in the form of serpiginous ulceration, lupus differs by its slower course, shallower and less painful ulcers, clean, soft, red base of granulation tissue, and by the presence in most cases of 'apple-jelly' spots near the ulcerating surface. The failure of specific syphilitic treatment is also an important aid to diagnosis.

Epithelioma and rodent ulcer differ from it by reason of their greater hardness, by the induration of the margin, and by the fact that they never appear in childhood, and rarely till after thirty, whereas lupus, though it may recur later, usually appears for the first time in early life.

From lupus erythematosus lupus vulgaris differs so much in appearance, in typical cases, that no mistake can be made. When the two forms occur in combination in the same individual, the 'apple-jelly' spots of vulgaris, and the hyperæmic follicles, with thin scales and sebaceous plugs of the erythematous variety, can usually be recognised.

Prognosis.—Lupus vulgaris affecting the skin is not in itself dangerous to life, although the attacks of erysipelas which occasionally complicate it may be serious. It sometimes disappears spontaneously and never recurs, and the diseased patches of tissue can be destroyed by energetic treatment. It is difficult, however, to do this effectually without damaging the skin so deeply as to cause subsequent cicatricial contraction, and hence, after all attempts to remove the diseased tissue alone, leaving the unaffected skin as little as possible damaged, the growth is prone to recur. Lupus erythematosus, except in the acute general form and when complicated with erysipelas, is also a benign disease.

The discoid is more amenable to treatment than the aggregated form, and the growth, when once destroyed, is less likely to recur than in lupus vulgaris.

Morbid Anatomy. Lupus vulgaris.—According to Friedländer and Thoma, whose observations have been confirmed in this country by Dr. Thin, lupus vulgaris begins by an aggregation of small round cells in the adventitia of the vessels of the corium. Local enlargements of the cellular deposit produce the little, scattered, roundish nodules, arranged like nests in fibrous loculi in the corium, composed of small young cells in a delicate fibrous network, permeated by a few dilated capillaries, and containing sometimes giant cells. The surrounding corium tissue remains at first free from infiltration, but the small-celled growth, extending along the vessels, reaches on one side the subpapillary layer and papillæ, and on the other the subcutaneous connective tissue and fat. The cellular infiltration next diffuses itself from these foci, till the whole corium, from the papillæ to the subcutaneous fat, is pervaded with small round cells, specially dense round the vessels, and hence accumulated thickly round the sweat glands, sebaceous and hair follicles. The cells of the glands and hair follicles, at first swollen and granular, soon degenerate and finally become atrophied and destroyed.

The rete Malpighii, at first normal, becomes later on thickened, and by the cellular infiltration, indistinguishable from the papillæ, its cells are swollen, more granular, and proliferating, and numerous round cells are scattered amongst them.

Fatty degeneration, breaking down of the cells, and ulceration of the growths next set in, but the process is a slow and superficial one, and the cells, in the deeper layers of an ulcerating spot, are frequently quite free from granules, and have distinct nuclei, while those on the surface are quite degenerated. Cicatrisation finally occurs, and smooth scars result, from which the hair follicles and glands are absent.

Lupus erythematosus.—In sections of the early 'primary eruptive spots' of the disease, the first changes which have been observed are dilatation of the vessels round the sebaceous glands and hair follicles, with slight œdema, and, when the spots are superficial, similar appearances in the adjacent papillæ. In the next stage the connective tissue immediately around the glands is found thickly infiltrated with round cells, which extend into the corium and papillæ, obscuring the connective-tissue bundles and the boundary between rete and papillæ; these, as atrophy begins, become cloudy, granular, and opaque, and begin to break down. The sweat glands are also sometimes affected.

Atrophy, or ulceration, with cicatrisation being completed, the hairs and glands are found degenerated, the connective tissue thickened, indurated, and obscured by fatty globules, and the atrophied blood vessels may be indicated only by pigmented strands. The rete is thinned, the papillæ absent, flattened, or wasted, and the whole corium is denser and has its meshes thickened.

Occasionally the granulation tissue, instead of spreading in lines along the meshes of the corium, becomes aggregated in nests, producing nodules identical with those of lupus vulgaris.

The painful nodes and swellings met with sometimes in acute outbreaks are due to inflammatory œdema of the skin and subcutaneous tissue.

Treatment.—Under the head of general treatment, applicable to both lupus erythematosus and lupus vulgaris, the chief indications are—first, if the general health is lowered, to restore and maintain it by means of a nutritious diet, with a moderate amount of stimulants and tonics, such as iron, quinine, &c.; and, secondly, to combat and remove, as far as possible, any morbid diathesis, such as the strumous or tubercular, with cod-liver oil, phosphate of lime, and iodide of iron. It should, however, be clearly understood that the administration of these remedies will not by itself remove the disease, for which purpose local treatment must be adopted.

In *lupus erythematosus* the local treatment consists in—

1. Removal of scales or crusts, if present.
2. Application of soothing remedies when the disease is in the acute stage.
3. Destruction of the new growth by mechanical or chemical means.

1. The removal of all crusts or scales, by careful oiling and washing with soap and water, is essential as a preliminary measure.
2. Simple ointments, such as vaseline ℥j with liq. plumbi ℳxxx, oleate of zinc or bismuth ℨiv to vaseline ℥j, zinc ointment, cold cream, cod-liver oil, sedative lotions containing

calamine, or glycerine and prussic acid, will be found useful. Mr. Hutchinson has seen great improvement follow the steady use of an ointment of liq. carbonis detergens ʒss to vaseline ʒj. All conditions that may irritate the skin, such as the heat of the sun, wind, or excessive cold, should be avoided.

3. For the destruction of the new growths, repeated multiple puncture, or linear scarification, as first recommended by Mr. Balmanno Squire, proves often of great service, destroying the dilated vessels and a portion of the new growth, which is still further removed by the subsequent inflammation. In very obstinate cases, where there is a more abundant formation of granulation tissue, scooping out the nodules with Volkmann's spoon may be necessary. Numerous caustics have been used, of which the spiritus saponatus alkalinus of Hebra is one of the best. It should be rubbed well into the patches with lint, removing all the scales. Crusts of dried-up blood and serum following the application should be removed by oiling, and the remedy used repeatedly till all traces of the disease have disappeared. Soft soap or liquor potassæ may be applied in the same way. Acids, such as the acid nitrate of mercury or nitric acid, may also be used, but are less effective than alkalies, as, owing to the fatty crusts, they often operate less upon the diseased parts than upon adjacent healthy tissue. Hebra's arsenical paste is of value when other measures fail ; its chief advantage is that it acts exclusively on the diseased tissue, and is not liable to cause toxic symptoms of absorption. It should be spread on lint and reapplied every twenty-four hours for two or three days. The severe pain and œdema of the skin, arising under its use, usually subsides in a few days, and the destroyed patches of growth desquamate, leaving small cavities, which soon heal.

In *lupus vulgaris* the use of sedatives is also indicated, if there be much irritability or inflammation.

The nodules of growth may be destroyed by (1) mechanical means, (2) the actual cautery, (3) chemical caustics.

For the first purpose Squire's linear scarification is suitable, but only for the milder and more superficial forms of lupus, as it does not penetrate deep enough to destroy the little nests which lie in the substance of the corium. Multiple puncture, by making, with a small sharp-pointed knife, numerous little stabs close to one another in the diseased nodules, frequently yields good results, especially when the nodules are small, isolated, and penetrate deeply into the true skin. Where the growth occurs in the form of a large plaque, it is necessary to remove it by means of Volkmann's spoon. The scraping should be done vigorously, and, as there is a marked difference between the soft, friable lupus tissue and the dense, fibrous corium, even on the face there need be no fear of doing it to excess. The edges of the patch especially should be thoroughly well scraped, and, after wiping the surface dry, any little masses of growth, lying in 'pockets' of the corium, should be scooped out or cauterised. When the crusts of dried blood and serum have separated, the patch will be found greatly diminished in size, and often entirely removed. The scrapings should be repeated from time to time till the growth is completely eradicated.

The actual cautery, as the galvanic wire or cone, the benzo-line cautery, or hot iron, may be used to destroy the growth, preferably when it occurs in confluent patches on the trunk and parts where scars are of little importance, and on the mucous membranes. The growth should be thoroughly ploughed up by the wire or cone, the resistance of the healthy tissue indicating when all the soft lupus deposit has been traversed; oil should be subsequently applied, and should any re-formation be observed after separation of the eschar and cicatrisation, it should be again destroyed. Paquelin's thermocautère is a most useful instrument for this purpose.

Of chemical caustics Hebra's arsenical paste, applied in the same way as in lupus erythematosus, and nitrate of silver in points bored into the nodules, are the best applications for dis-seminated patches. Potassa fusa, in stick or solution, or chloride of zinc paste, or acids, such as strong nitric acid, acid nitrate of mercury, or carbolic acid, are all valuable, and have been found efficacious in different cases.

RHINOSCLEROMA.

Definition.—A peculiar affection, of extremely chronic course, consisting in the formation, on the skin or mucous membrane around the anterior nares, of dense roundish tubercles, which have no tendency to ulcerate or undergo retrogression.

Symptoms.—An abstract of the description of Kaposi, based on fifteen cases, is as follows :—The tubercles, isolated or conglomerate, are either smooth, supple, and the same colour as the normal skin, or bright or brownish red and glossy. The epidermis over them is cracked and fissured, and from the rhagades a viscid secretion, drying into yellowish scabs, exudes. The nodules are somewhat elastic, seem cartilaginous to the touch, and are painful on pressure ; they are embedded in the skin, which is normal at their margins.

The nodule, beginning slowly as a thickening and induration of the skin on the septum or edge of one of the alæ, extends gradually into the meatus, which it greatly narrows, to the cheek, and to the upper lip, and causes great deformity.

Diagnosis.—1. From a syphilitic gumma it is distinguished by the extremely chronic course, absence of degeneration or ulceration, obstinate resistance to treatment, and the peculiar localisation and restriction of the disease.

2. If the tumour be prominent, glistening, and covered with dilated vessels, it can be diagnosed from keloid only by the history and by microscopical examination.

Prognosis.—Though rhinoscleroma absolutely resists treatment, it is not fatal to life, and is not liable to grow rapidly, affect the constitution, or undergo ulceration. The deformity and the obstruction to the nares are the chief inconveniences arising from it.

Morbid Anatomy.—According to Kaposi, who has described the disease at length, the nodule, which cuts easily, presents on section a pale red, granular surface, bleeding moderately. Microscopically the epidermis is found normal, the papillæ somewhat longer and club-shaped, and their tissue and that of the corium replaced by a delicately fibrillated, small-meshed network, enclosing numerous small round cells and pervaded by a few small vessels. The growth, which somewhat resembles lymphoid tissue, is most abundant in the papillary layer, but extends to the deeper layers of the corium, and sometimes even to the cartilage. The hair follicles and root sheaths embedded in the growth are normal.

Treatment.—Excision of the growth has hitherto been followed by recurrence, and all internal or local applications fail to remove it.

Of Vessels.

1. Nævus.   2. Angioma.

NÆVUS.

Definition.—Is a spot limited to one or other region of the body, light bluish or dark red in colour, composed usually of dilated capillaries and veins, congenital or appearing shortly after birth.

Symptoms.—Nævi may be smooth and level with, or only slightly raised above, the general surface, or tuberculated, with irregular prominences on the surface. They may affect merely the superficial layers of the skin, or extend throughout its whole thickness, and even into the subcutaneous tissue. They can be emptied of blood by pressure, the superficial varieties becoming pale and the nodular loose and flaccid, but the blood soon returns on removing the compression, and they resume their normal tint. They occur most commonly on the face, scalp, and neck, but they may be met with on the arms and trunk, and but rarely on the lower extremities.

Diagnosis.—Nævi can only be mistaken, immediately after birth, for the small bruises caused by forceps, but an interval of a week will decide the question.

Prognosis.—Nævi tend to grow slowly, and when composed

of large vessels and ulceration takes place, serious hæmorrhage may be the result.

Morbid Anatomy.—A nævus consists of an aggregation of dilated blood vessels, the walls of which are sometimes thickened, and the plexuses do not correspond with the normal meshwork of the part.

Treatment.—No satisfactory mode of treating the superficial nævi has been introduced, but those most usually employed are strong acids or the actual cautery. Both of these always leave a scar, but the latter is probably the best.

ANGIOMA.

Definition.—A new growth composed of dilated vessels, closely applied to one another, arising usually in the subcutaneous tissue, and sometimes in the skin, and not congenital.

Symptoms.—Angiomata may arise as little slightly raised spots, of a bright red colour, resembling nævi, but differing from them in being developed in adult life instead of being congenital. When arising in the subcutaneous tissue, the skin, at first freely movable over them, becomes gradually involved, and they then appear as bluish-red tumours, much like nodular nævi. The growths may be single or multiple, and often cause pain from pressure on nerves.

Morbid Anatomy.—Sections of the tumours show large roundish or oval spaces filled with blood, and limited by delicate connective-tissue trabeculæ lined by an endothelium. A kind of capsule frequently surrounds the growth.

Treatment.—If the size and situation be inconvenient, and hæmorrhage and pain result, it may be enucleated. It does not usually recur.

Lymphatic-tissue New Growths.

LYMPHANGIOMA.

Tumours composed of dilated lymphatic vessels, or of lymphatic glands which have undergone cystic degeneration, are occasionally met with. As a rule they do not implicate the corium primarily, and belong to the domain of general surgery rather than to that of diseases of the skin.

In a case described by Kaposi, under the name of lymphangioma tuberosum multiplex, hundreds of small, rounded, brownish, slightly raised nodules were found embedded in the substance of the corium. They were about the size of lentils, became pale on pressure, and were slightly painful. On microscopic examination of an excised tubercle it was found to consist of circular or oval spaces, most numerous in the deeper layers of the corium, lined by endothelium, and identical in structure with dilated lymphatics. No changes were found in the blood vessels or papillary layer, and, with the exception of pigmentation of the lower rete cells, the epidermis was normal.

The tumours exercised no influence on the general health, gave rise to no subjective symptoms, and extended but slowly; they showed no tendency to involution, and remained unaffected by treatment.

CHAPTER XX.

Sub-class B.—*Malignant.*

Lepra maculosa, tuberosa, anæsthetica—Carcinoma—Epithelioma—
Ulcus rodens—Sarcoma.

LEPRA—LEPROSY.

Definition.—A chronic constitutional disease, characterised by the development of small-celled nodular growths in the skin, mucous membranes, and nerves.

Symptoms.—Leprosy, formerly prevalent throughout the whole of Europe, and still occurring endemically on the west coast of Norway and on the shores of the Mediterranean, is now met with in this country only in sporadic cases. The persons attacked or their immediate progenitors have usually resided in countries where the disease is endemic, and the tendency to its development is hereditary. Opinions are still divided as to whether it is contagious; it is possible, however, that the secretions of a person affected with the disease may at some period or other be capable of communicating it to others. Though no primary lesion, analogous to the hard chancre of syphilis, is known to occur in leprosy, the disease frequently arises, and runs a typical course several years after the person attacked has left an infected locality, and though no morbid phenomena, resembling those of infantile syphilis, may be present at or soon after birth, in the children they may develope leprosy after an interval of many years, without ever having been exposed to the conditions supposed to give rise to it. Dr. Liveing is of opinion that many instances in which the disease is thought to have

Q

arisen spontaneously in this country are possibly due to an un-traceable hereditary taint. Mr. Hutchinson considers that a diet composed chiefly of fish favours the development of leprosy.

The disease usually begins by a *prodromal stage*, absent or very slight in some cases, during which no characteristic symptoms of leprosy are present. Malaise, languor and depression, gastric disturbance, and sometimes slight shivering and evening pyrexia, may last for months or even years. Finally, the phenomena peculiar to the disease make their appearance, and, according to the most prominent symptoms present, three varieties are described—lepra maculosa, tuberosa, and anæsthetica. They differ in degree rather than in kind, and sometimes the characteristics of one variety are present together with those peculiar to another.

Leprosy affects both sexes equally, and though most frequent in early adult life, it is met with at all ages. The macular and tubercular forms are the most common in temperate climates, while the anæsthetic variety predominates in the tropics.

LEPRA MACULOSA.

After a prodromal stage of varying duration, maculæ, at first pale red and later dark brown or reddish grey, appear on various parts of the surface. They are smooth, glistening, flat or only slightly elevated, present defined or somewhat indistinct outlines, and vary from a half to three lines in diameter. The affected patches of skin, thickened, indurated, and somewhat tender on pressure, enlarge gradually at their margins, which are dark reddish-brown in colour, while at their centre they become paler. They are largest and most numerous on the trunk, limbs, and sometimes on the palms and soles also, but are less marked on the face. Occasionally in the earlier stages of the disease the patches undergo complete involution, leaving the skin normal in colour or white, smooth, and glistening. After existing in this form for years, during which the patches appear and disappear at intervals, with little or no constitutional disturbance, symptoms characteristic of the anæsthetic or tuberous varieties become superadded, and the disease assumes graver features.

LEPRA TUBEROSA.

After a *prodromal* and a *macular* stage the smooth brownish infiltrated patches become more prominent, and cover a larger surface. Small round tubercles, varying in size from a shot to a small nut, next make their appearance in the centre of the macular elevations or in healthy skin. They are smooth or covered by fissured cuticle, reddish brown in colour, with ramifying vessels on the surface, and are firm and somewhat tender on pressure. The natural prominences of the skin and its furrows become exaggerated, and the face presents a prematurely aged, a sad, and morose expression. It is also broader and quadrangular in shape, brownish red and glazed in appearance. The eyebrows are more prominent, and are bald except at their outer angles, and the nose, cheeks, chin, and lips are affected with several tubercles, which give them a thickened, irregular appearance, and produce a ' pouting expression' of mouth, resembling that of a mulatto. This characteristic alteration of the whole countenance is termed ' facies leontina.'

Similar large infiltrated patches and aggregations of tubercles are met with on the body and extremities. The hands and feet become greatly deformed, the nails are cracked and distorted, the hair and sebaceous glands on the patches and tubercles atrophy and disappear, and, owing to the pain and tenderness in the soles, walking becomes impossible. Chronic œdema of the legs, producing a condition of elephantiasis, is usually met with in cases of long standing. After some time the mucous membrane of the mouth, the pharynx, &c., are occupied by similar tubercles, which, like the rest, may, at the commencement of the disease, have undergone involution and atrophy, leaving roundish depressed and deeply pigmented patches, and in the latter stages, becoming obstinate, may last, with little or no change, for years. They may also give rise to abscesses, which slowly discharge their

contents, or on slight irritation undergo sloughing and ulceration, which in the hands and feet may cause necrosis of the bones
or openings in the joints, and lead to the loss of fingers or toes.

At this stage more or less fever, with rigors and severe
depression, is usually present, and in acute cases the super-
vention of pneumonia, pleurisy, diarrhœa, or other internal
complications may rapidly prove fatal. In more chronic cases
the above symptoms gradually recede, and there may be an
interval of comparative comfort, during which the disease remains
stationary or progresses only slowly. Recurring periods of febrile
exacerbations, with more extension and rapid development and
ulceration of the tubercles, progressively lower the general health,
and may induce a condition of great prostration and marasmus,
which ultimately causes death. Very frequently, however, after
the disease in the tubercular form has lasted for some years, the
symptoms of anæsthetic leprosy may set in and gradually become
predominant.

LEPRA ANÆSTHETICA.

After a prodromal stage, characterised frequently by the
periodic appearance of bullæ, resembling those of pemphigus, or
sometimes of maculæ, during which the general health presents
little or no change, the anæsthetic variety becomes developed.
Patches of variable extent and situation on normal skin, as well
as on that which is the seat of macular infiltration or has been
previously attacked by bullæ, are found to be hyperæsthetic.
Any attempt, therefore, to walk, grasp, or to use the hands excites
painful or burning sensations or reflex spasmodic movements,
and numbness and tingling in the extremities may also exist.
Various subcutaneous nerves—the ulnar, radial, median, peroneal,
&c.—present extremely painful nodular enlargements. After a
variable period, the hyperæsthetic parts gradually become less
irritable and anæsthesia commences in the previously sensitive
patches or in places where some abnormal pigmentation has
existed. A pinkish hyperæsthetic zone usually surrounds the
anæsthetic area, in which sensibility to pain, to touch, to heat

or cold, or to electricity, may be modified, and in the later stages wholly absent. During the course of the disease, as well as in the prodromal stage, bullæ may appear. Atrophy of the skin and of the muscles supplied by the affected nerves next sets in, and in consequence various paralytic deformities of the hands and feet are produced. Constant chilliness is complained of, and the temperature of the body is much diminished. Either spontaneously or on slight irritation, of which there is no consciousness on account of the loss of sensation, ulceration of the skin takes place at the extremities, opening the joints and leading to the separation of one or more fingers or toes; hence this variety has been called *lepra mutilans*. Necrosis and caries of the bones and moist or dry gangrene of the extremities, attended with severe constitutional symptoms, are also liable to occur without obvious cause. Towards the termination of the disease, marasmus, diarrhœa, or clonic and tetanic spasms set in, ultimately causing death.

Diagnosis.—A well-marked attack of leprosy, with the characteristic pigmentation and appearance of face, cannot be confused with any other disease. In milder forms, however, leprosy may be mistaken for pemphigus, leucoderma, lupus, or syphilis.

The bullous eruption of leprosy differs from pemphigus in that the blebs are solitary or few in number, and usually associated with the anæsthetic patches.

For diagnosis from leucoderma see p. 199.

When the tubercles of leprosy are arranged in aggregated patches or in small nodules round a cicatricial centre, there is much resemblance to lupus. The firmer, more persistent character of the nodules, which are not soft and like 'apple jelly,' as in lupus, their tenderness on pressure, and the glistening, oily look of the infiltrated skin in leprosy are the chief points of diagnosis between them.

At an early stage of the disease, if the maculæ are small, pinkish, and fade on pressure or present a small central tubercle, there is a resemblance to a papulo-macular syphilide. The spots of leprosy are, however, usually larger, even to the full size of the palm, an appearance never seen in syphilis; they are more infiltrated and tender on pressure, are more persistent, and change to a dark-brown or white colour, remaining smooth and shining instead of acquiring scales, crusts, &c., or forming serpiginous ulcers. The 'facies leontina' is also characteristic of leprosy.

Prognosis.—Leprosy, though usually chronic, is almost always a fatal disease, and only a few cases are recorded of complete recovery, most so-called cures being merely periods of remission, in which the symptoms remain in abeyance or undergo some retrogression, but after a longer or shorter period resume their former course. The tubercular form lasts a shorter time than the other varieties, its average duration being eight or ten years, while anæsthetic leprosy may be prolonged for twenty years. Occasionally tubercular leprosy, when once fully developed, runs an acute course, being attended with much fever and rapid evolution and disintegration of new tubercles, and then the disease progresses in a few months to a stage which it would usually have reached only after years.

Morbid Anatomy.—Vertical sections through the cutaneous nodules show reddish granular masses, limited by a fibrous capsule or shading off gradually into the corium, which extend sometimes close to the epidermis and at other times invade the subcutaneous tissue. Under the microscope they are seen to consist of small round or spindle-shaped cells, which in young nodules are most abundant round the thick-walled vessels and the plexuses of the sweat and sebaceous glands and of the hair follicles, while in the older ones they are densely aggregated, and lie in the delicate meshwork derived from the fibres of the corium. Their central parts contain no vessels ; the papillæ are obliterated, the cuticle thinned, and the glands and hairs atrophied or degenerated, but a rich vascular network is formed in the margins. The cells of the new growth have distinct nuclei, and their protoplasm presents a somewhat cloudy 'ground-glass' appearance ; globules are found here and there, and the arrectores pilorum are said to be hypertrophied. A very slight cellular infiltration has been found in parts which presented the appearance of discoloration or pinkish maculæ.

The morbid changes in the nerves—*neuritis leprosa*—are as follows :—At points exposed to pressure, or where the nerve is near the surface, its trunk presents fusiform enlargements, greyish or yellowish, semi-translucent, sometimes even brown or blackish in appearance, and it is much firmer than when normal. Transverse sections show the general nerve sheath unaltered, except that its vessels are slightly thickened. Beneath the funicular sheaths, which are usually somewhat thickened and in old-standing cases sclerosed, aggregations of small cells of the same nature as those composing the cutaneous nodules are found, compressing the nerve fibrils and sending cords of cells in between them. More or less fatty degeneration and disintegration of the medullary sheaths, and in later stages complete atrophy of the nerve fibrils, next takes place, and the hyperæsthesia at first produced by the irritation of the nerves owing to the growth gives place to anæsthesia as they become destroyed. In the affected portions of nerves, as well as the skin in which they are distributed, Dr. Vandyke Carter has found roundish or oval brown pigmented bodies. Pigmentation and thickening of the vessels in the cerebral and spinal pia mater, as well as albuminous-looking deposits in the meninges and degenerative changes in the spinal cord, have been described by Danielssen and Boeck, but have not been met with by Dr. Carter in India.

Treatment.—This must be directed to the improvement of the general health by nutritious diet, tonics, good hygienic conditions, cleanliness, exercise, and removal from districts where the disease is endemic. Internal remedies, of which many have from time to time been vaunted as specifics, have little or no influence on the general malady. Cod-liver oil, internally and by inunction, chaulmoogra oil or gurjun balsam applied in the same way, and the local stimulation of the deposits by the inunction of cashew oil, iodine, &c., are sometimes attended with benefit. Ulcers should be treated on general principles, and the hyperæsthesia relieved by opiates.

In the quiescent intervals galvanism is often useful in the treatment of paralysis and muscular atrophy.

CARCINOMA CUTIS.

Definition.—A malignant growth in the skin, composed of nests of cells contained in an alveolar stroma, occurring in the form of nodules which spread by infiltration of the surrounding tissues, affect the adjacent lymphatic glands, recur after removal, and prove fatal by ulceration, cachexia, and exhaustion.

Symptoms.—Carcinoma of the skin is usually secondary to the development of the disease in other organs; it affects the cutis by continuous extension from the deeper parts, or occurs in the form of isolated nodules, usually multiple, beginning either in the subcutaneous connective tissue and soon involving the corium or arising primarily in the latter. Structurally it presents sometimes the characters of scirrhus, sometimes those of encephaloid cancer.

In scirrhus of the breast, as the disease extends towards the surface, the skin becomes adherent to the tumour, drawn in at the centre, indurated, and infiltrated. The margin is often raised into reddish-brown, elastic nodules, and similar masses may develope in the vicinity of, but not in visible continuity with, the primary growth. Occasionally, when scirrhus affects the liver or stomach, numerous small roundish or oval, firm, and painful nodules may occur in the substance of the corium, which present the same structure as the original mass. If life be sufficiently prolonged, like the nodules in scirrhus mammæ, they gradually extend to the surface, break down, and form excavated ulcers with everted indurated edges, a sloughy firm base, and foul ichorous discharge.

Carcinoma encephaloides occurs sometimes primarily in the skin as a rare affection in old persons. Multiple nodular masses of various sizes, most numerous on the face and hands and of a dark red colour, are present over the whole surface. They soon break down and acquire a greenish, firm crust or slough, producing excavated ulcers like those of scirrhus, which tend to spread in all directions. The lymphatic glands and internal organs are less liable to secondary infection than in scirrhus.

Diagnosis.—Multiple scirrhus nodules may be mistaken for those of fibroma; their hard, painful nature, their rapid growth and tendency to break-down if life lasts long enough, the presence usually of a primary spot of disease in some other organ, and the microscopical structure of one of the nodules, will be sufficient for diagnosis.

From gummata they are distinguished by the absence of a history or of other evidences of syphilis, by their great firmness, and by their structure. Encephaloid nodules growing rapidly, and forming ulcers with indurated, everted edges, can hardly be mistaken for any other disease.

Prognosis.—Both forms of carcinoma are invariably fatal.

Morbid Anatomy.—Scirrhus of the skin presents the same structure as in other organs of the body, and consists of nests of small roundish or polygonal cells contained in alveoli, the walls of which are comparatively thick and firm. As the edges of the tumour, the alveolar structure gradually passes into that of the normal tissue, which is very thickly infiltrated with round cells. In encephaloid the cells are larger, contain large round nuclei with clear protoplasm surrounding them, and the alveoli are composed of thin septa of connective tissue. The blood vessels are larger and more freely distributed than in scirrhus; their walls are thin and cavernous, and dilatations and hæmorrhages are frequent.

Treatment.—This can only be palliative. The strength should be supported by nutritious food and stimulants, the pain relieved by opiates, and the ulcers dressed with astringent and antiseptic lotions.

EPITHELIOMA CUTIS.

Definition.—A malignant new growth of the skin, infiltrating the tissues and spreading along the lymphatics to the glands, characterised by a tendency to local recurrence after removal and by slight liability to the formation of the secondary growths in distant parts.

Symptoms.—Epithelioma occurs but rarely under forty, and is most commonly met with on the lower lip, the external genitals, and the face. It begins as small rounded, isolated or aggregated nodules embedded in the substance of the skin, which in the course of months or years enlarge and form a roundish, buttonlike mass, raised slightly above the surface of the skin, with defined sloping edges and a smooth or somewhat irregular warty-looking surface. The little tumour is yellowish or brownish in colour, and covered with ramifying vessels, is extremely hard, usually somewhat painful, and, though at first freely movable, becomes at a later stage adherent to the deeper structures. The surface next desquamates, becomes excoriated, and is covered with a thin, adherent, brownish scab in its centre, under which is found a reddish ulcer with a granular base and slight sticky secretion. The edges are prominent, everted, indurated, irregular, and often present little translucent, rounded, vesicular-looking nodules towards their outer margin. Infiltration, followed by ulceration, goes on in all directions; the neighbouring lymphatic glands become enlarged, nodular, and indurated, and often break down to form malignant ulcers; and severe lancinating pains are usually present, with wasting and much prostration. On the scrotum the disease usually begins as an irregular, warty mass, frequently pigmented, which becomes excoriated on the surface, and then gives rise to sloughy ulcers. On the lip it often begins as a persistent fissure, covered by a thin scab, and at first without any induration of the surrounding tissues; but the base gradually becomes hard, the margins prominent and infiltrated, till a typical ulcer is finally produced.

Diagnosis.—Epithelioma may be mistaken for syphilis, lupus, or a simple excoriated wart. The age, the previous history and course of the affection, the pain, which is usually greater than in syphilis, and occasionally the detection under the microscope of epithelial 'globes' in the scrapings of the ulcers, will aid the diagnosis from syphilis, and when a hard, translucent edge or small, clear, marginal nodules are present the distinction is easy.

For diagnosis from lupus see p. 216.

An abraded wart cannot in many cases be distinguished from a commencing epithelioma, more especially since epithelioma not unfrequently attacks a wart which has lasted for some time. The persistence and the slowness of the ulcerated surface to heal point towards epithelioma.

Prognosis.—In the early stages epithelioma, if completely destroyed, may not recur, but if considerable infiltration of the tissue and glandular affection have set in, the disease will return after excision or cauterisation, and will ultimately prove fatal.

Morbid Anatomy.—Vertical sections through a mass of epithelioma have a whitish, granular appearance, and are firm and friable. Under the microscope, at the margin of the growth the interpapillary processes of the rete are seen to be enlarged, much elongated, and pressing on the papillæ, which, towards the centre portion of the growth, are reduced to thin, fibrous septa. The epithelial cylinders, composed of spinous rete cells with a few scattered leucocytes, contain here and there rounded masses of flattened, laminated cells, resembling the transverse section of an onion, which are called the epidermic 'globes' or 'pearls.' They extend into the corium, which is more vascular and infiltrated with numerous small cells, denser near the epithelium. The blood vessels, at first numerous in the connective-tissue processes between the epithelial cylinders, become gradually pressed upon and obliterated by them, which causes the superficial and older portions of the nodule to break down and ulcerate. In sections parallel to surface epithelial growths, as was first shown by Köster, are seen filling the lymphatics, and in this way the glands become 'infected' and the seats of secondary epithelial deposits. The sebaceous and sweat glands and the hair follicles involved in the growth show signs of epithelial proliferation, followed by degeneration, and are ultimately destroyed.

Treatment.—A thorough removal of the growth by free excision or its complete destruction by caustics are the only measures which give any hope of a cure.

As caustics potassa fusa, Vienna paste, chloride of zinc, and Hebra's arsenical paste are the most suitable.

The disease in most cases recurs, and repeated operations or cauterisations, though they only temporarily check the progress of the disease, give some intervals of comparative comfort and prolong life.

ULCUS RODENS.

Rodent ulcer is considered by most Continental dermatologists to be merely a variety of epithelioma, and several English observers have found the growth to present the microscopic structure of the latter disease; it presents, however, certain clinical characters that require a separate description.

Symptoms.—It begins as a small, smooth, pale papule or tubercle, situated usually on the upper half of the face; it gradually increases in size, and, after lasting perhaps for many years, commences to ulcerate. An ulcer, with hard, sinuous edges, often irregular in outline, and attended with little or no pain, but extending gradually in depth and area, is thus produced. Its base is said to be not granulated, but smooth, glassy, and dull reddish yellow in appearance, and as the margin extends cicatrisation occasionally takes place in the centre. Slowly invading the deeper parts, ulceration may expose even the bones of the face, but there is never any secondary glandular infiltration, and the general health is little affected. It occurs in persons past middle age, and usually in those advanced in life.

Diagnosis.—The main differences from ordinary epithelioma consist in the extreme chronic, painless course, the absence of glandular infiltration and cachexia, the tendency in some cases to cicatrisation, and the less marked liability to recurrence if the disease be once thoroughly destroyed.

Treatment.—Complete destruction of the growth at an early stage by excision, by scraping, or by caustics, will often cure, and in all cases much retard the progress of the disease.

SARCOMA CUTIS.

Definition.—Sarcoma of the skin is a rare affection, occurring primarily in the corium and subsequently to the origin of the disease in some other situation.

Symptoms.—Small rounded reddish, or bluish-brown nodules, varying in size from a small shot to a hazel nut, appear at first on the feet or hands, and then scattered over the whole surface of the body. They are isolated, smooth, and elastic to the touch, and in a late stage of the disease break down and slough. The disease occurs most frequently in males and in persons over forty years of age.

Diagnosis.—It differs from carcinoma in beginning most commonly in the feet, in the absence of alveolar structure, and in the general freedom from implication of the lymphatic glands.

Prognosis.—Death usually occurs within two or three years from the commencement, probably owing to the existence of similar tumours in the vital organs.

Morbid Anatomy.—The nodules, when examined under the microscope, are seen to consist of round or spindle-shaped pigmented cells, traversed by thin-walled, cavernous vessels, and often presenting patches of hæmorrhagic infiltration and degeneration.

Treatment.—As in carcinoma of the skin, this can be only palliative.

DIVISION II.—DISEASES OF THE APPENDAGES OF THE SKIN.

CHAPTER XXI.

SUBDIVISION A.—*Of the Sebaceous Glands.*

Seborrhœa, oleosa sicca, Ichthyosis sebacea neonatorum—Acne punctata, comedo, milium—Acne vulgaris—Acne sycosis—Acne rosacea —Molluscum contagiosum.

SUBDIVISION B.—*Of the Sweat Glands.*

Hyperidrosis—Anidrosis—Bromidrosis—Chromidrosis—Sudamina.

SUBDIVISION A.—*Of the Sebaceous Glands.*

SEBORRHŒA—ACNE SEBACEA.

Definition.—Seborrhœa is a condition due to increased secretion of the sebaceous glands, in which the sebum mixed with dirt accumulates on otherwise healthy skin.

Before describing the different varieties of seborrhœa it will be well to discuss briefly the composition of sebum and how it is produced. Kölliker shows that the sebaceous glands are constantly giving off cells, which, when first formed at the bottom of the glands, are pale and only slightly granular, but which, when they are forced to the surface by the formation of fresh cells, become filled with a quantity of fat granules. These granules at a later stage coalesce into a single globule, and the wall of the cell becomes stronger and more horny. Seborrhœa consists in the increased production of these oil globules, and may be divided into three varieties—S. oleosa, S. sicca, and ichthyosis sebacea neonatorum.

Symptoms.—*Seborrhœa oleosa* occurs usually between the ages of fifteen and twenty-five, and affects the cheeks, nose, and forehead. The exudation of oil from the sebaceous glands gives a greasy appearance to the skin, which next becomes dirty, owing to the liability of the oil to attract and absorb particles of dust and dirt floating in the air. When this condition has lasted for some time crusts are formed, which may vary greatly in colour, and when they are raised small processes of sebum can be drawn from the follicles. When the disease occurs on hairy places the hair becomes matted, in consequence of which dirt adheres and vermin accumulate, constituting the condition known as *plica Polonica.*

S. oleosa also occurs on the genitals of both sexes, and is known as *smegma præputii et clitoridis.* When neglected it forms thin crusts, which in the male are situated on the glans penis beneath the prepuce, and in the female around the clitoris and in the neighbouring grooves. If allowed to remain untouched for a long time, they cause severe local irritation and inflammation, a condition which may be mistaken for gonorrhœa. *Vernix caseosa* is a name given by Hebra to a similar deposit over the whole body of new-born infants.

Seborrhœa sicca is produced in asimilar way to S. oleosa, but gives rise to the formation either of a dry, light yellow crust or a branny coating to the skin. The regions most usually affected are the scalp and other hairy parts of the body. Scales of epidermis and dried sebum, which are constantly being formed and ought to be removed, are, owing to a want of cleanliness, allowed to accumulate in the hair, and are known as scurf. The affection does not last long without injuring the hair itself, which gradually falls off and is replaced by badly developed hair till partial baldness is the result. When the disease is of long standing further changes take place in the scalp, and itching, which is absent in the earlier stage of the disease, may eventually arise from an eczematous condition of the skin.

Ichthyosis sebacea neonatorum must not on account of its name be confused with true ichthyosis, but Hebra has thus termed the affection of new-born infants formerly known as ichthyosis congenita. The symptoms appear within a few hours of birth, when the skin presents a smooth, glossy, and somewhat purple appearance. It is also covered with a quantity of fissures, which are most numerous on the fingers and toes and over the flexures of the joints. The slightest movement causes pain, and in severe cases the child is unable to suck.

Diagnosis.—S. oleosa may be mistaken for lupus erythematosus, but greater swelling and redness, more adherent scales, and a tendency to scar are found in the latter.

S. sicca may be mistaken for three diseases when it attacks the scalp—eczema, psoriasis, and ringworm. For the diagnosis from the two former see table, p. 139. From ringworm it may be distinguished by the history of the case, the absence of short broken hairs, the greater difficulty in extracting the hairs, and by aid of the microscope.

Ichthyosis sebacea neonatorum may be distinguished from genuine ichthyosis by the fact that the former is local and not general.

Prognosis.—This depends on the cause of the condition, for when it occurs in the course of a serious disease the prognosis is unfavourable, while under suitable treatment recovery is in ordinary cases usually rapid.

Treatment.—Both local and constitutional means are used, but the former are the most important. In all varieties thorough cleanliness is necessary, and if crusts are formed they should be removed with oil, soft soap, or lard. After removal of the crusts the part should be dressed with a slightly stimulating ointment, such as zinc, weak carbolic acid, or tar, and in S. sicca of the scalp a lotion of borax is useful.

Internally tonics, such as arsenic, iron, and the mineral acids, should be administered in full and repeated doses.

ACNE PUNCTATA.

Definition.—A disease of the skin caused by the retention of sebum in the ducts of the sebaceous glands and hair follicles.

Acne punctata occurs in two forms, differing in colour, which are therefore respectively called *nigra* and *alba*, but are usually known as comedo and milium.

Symptoms.—*Comedones* usually occur between the ages of fourteen and twenty-five, and attack the face, chest, and back, in small black spots, which look, as Hebra suggests, like grains of gunpowder inserted into the skin. If one of these black spots be compressed between the nails, a long, wormlike body with a black head is forced out. The little mass thus ejected consists of retained sebum and the black head of dirt which has adhered to the cheesy material. The cavity from which the wormlike body is expressed is the neck of a hair follicle into which a sebaceous gland opens, and the wormlike appearance is caused by its shape. In the substance of the mass there is also, however, in some cases a living grub, which has nothing to do with the retention of the sebum and is quite as often found in normal glands. It is called the acarus folliculorum, and was first discovered by Henle in 1841.

Milium appears in the same situations as comedones, and at the same time of life, but often terminates in an inflammatory process, giving rise to acne vulgaris. It consists of a small swelling under the cuticle, which is caused by the retention of sebum in the sebaceous gland and not in the neck of the hair follicle, and is white in colour, owing to the impossibility of accumulating dirt, as in the comedones.

Diagnosis.—These varieties of acne punctata can only be mistaken for acne vulgaris, but the absence of redness and other inflammatory signs in them is sufficiently characteristic.

Prognosis.—It is perfectly harmless and easy to cure, but is liable to recur.

Morbid Anatomy.—On incising the skin over one of the fine

R

white granules in milium a small round body can be turned
out with the point of a needle, which on compression breaks up
into fine laminated scales. A thin vertical section examined
with the microscope shows a mass of horny epithelial cells, surrounding frequently a central space filled with broken-down
cells and fatty débris, and enclosed in a thin capsule of a finely
fibrillated connective tissue. The whole mass consists of an
altered sebaceous follicle, the cells of which, instead of undergoing fatty degeneration and alteration into sebum, have become
cornified. It is covered by the papillary layer of the corium,
which has to be cut through in order to remove it. Frequently
the little epidermic globule is fixed by a fine pedicle, consisting
of an atrophied hair follicle, to the corium.

Treatment.—For comedones thorough cleanliness and
friction of the part affected is the best treatment. The plugs
of sebum should be squeezed out with the finger nails or with a
watch key, and a mild stimulating ointment containing a small
quantity of sulphur or tar should be afterwards applied. The
skin over the little tumours in milium should be carefully divided
and the mass squeezed out. Constitutional remedies are necessary in both conditions if any functional irregularity can be
discovered.

ACNE VULGARIS.

Definition.—Acne vulgaris is a disease of the skin characterised by the appearance of nodules or pustules, caused by inflammation of the hair follicles and sebaceous glands.

Symptoms.—It occurs in the same places as A. punctata and
at the same time of life. It consists of comedones, which by their
presence or by local irritation lead to an inflammatory condition
of the gland, producing raised red pimples, varying in size from
a small seed to a pea. The disease is termed *A. indurata* if the
inflammation extends deeply into the skin, and *A. pustulosa* if
pus is formed. In the latter, after the pustule bursts or the retained matter is expelled, the spot disappears, but a small shallow

scar is left. If the disease attacks the forehead it is termed *A. frontalis*, and appears in the form of large papules, tubercles, or pustules, which leave scars when they are cured. At times, if the inflammation is severe, the disease resembles a boil. A severe form of A. vulgaris is produced by the local application of tar, and by the internal administration to susceptible persons of such drugs as iodide and bromide of potassium. The usual theories as to the cause of A. vulgaris—excessive venery, or the too free use of alcohol or highly seasoned food—are very doubtful, and its true cause is a matter of uncertainty. However, it is common in the scrofulous and tubercular diathesis.

Diagnosis.—Acne vulgaris is easily recognisable, but may be mistaken for small-pox in a certain stage (see p. 51) or for a syphilide. In the latter case some other syphilitic eruption at the same time is generally to be found (see A. syphilitica, p. 86).

Prognosis.—Acne vulgaris is never fatal, though it produces great annoyance to the individual, and in time the disease will disappear, for it rarely persists after twenty-five or twenty-six years of age.

Morbid Anatomy.—In A. vulgaris the sebaceous plug, blocking the excretory duct of the gland, acts as a foreign body and excites inflammatory hyperæmia, followed by serous exudation into and round the hair follicles and glands. If the plug be not removed, the further inflammation it excites gives rise to pus formation in and round the sebaceous glands, surrounded by firm, painful, inflammatory induration of the adjacent connective tissue, which subsequently becomes hypertrophied. In this way the hard tubercles of A. indurata are produced. The formation of pus is usually slight, and being at the closed extremity of the gland, is not near the surface but in the substance of the corium, and is therefore not usually seen until the nodule is incised or contents evacuated. When the pus is in excess or obviously near the surface, the condition known as A. pustulosa is produced.

Treatment.—The treatment should be both local and constitutional. Thorough sponging with hot water and friction are

R 2

of the greatest importance. The plugs of sebum should be removed by pressure, and the pus liberated by small incisions.
Soaps containing free alkali are of value, and Hebra's spiritus
saponatus alkalinus is one of the best forms. The part should
be well rubbed with it, but its use should not be prolonged over
more than a few days on account of the great irritation liable to
be produced. It is well also to apply ointments containing a
small quantity of sulphur and creosote, such as—

Sublimed sulphur, grs. 30; white precipitate, grs. 10; æthiops
mineral, grs. 10; olive oil, ℥ij; creosote, ♏iv; lard to ℥ix. (*Skin
Hospital*);

or lotions containing perchloride of mercury gr. ¼ or ½ to the ℥j.
While pustules are forming it is well to touch them lightly with
acid nitrate of mercury, taking care that the fluid does not run
on to the sound skin.

The constitutional treatment should consist of such remedies
as are calculated to maintain the general health by regulating
the various functions of the body. The diet should be carefully
attended to, and stimulants should be prohibited.

ACNE SYCOSIS—ACNE MENTAGRA.

Definition.—Hebra's definition is 'a disease of chronic
course, non-contagious, attacking the hairy parts of the cutaneous surface, and characterised by the development of papules
and tubercles, continuous thickenings, and pustules of various
sizes, all of these having invariably hairs passing through them.'

Symptoms.—Acne sycosis consists of a chronic inflammation
and suppuration of the hair follicles, and therefore attacks only
the hairy parts of the body, but the most usual site is the beard.
The cause often suggested for A. sycosis is the use of blunt
razors, but this is doubtful, since persons who never shave are
liable to it. The pimples first appear like those of A. vulgaris,
but with a hair passing through each of them, and as they get

larger and assume the character of tubercles they may coalesce and form a thick, indurated mass, limited entirely to the hairy region and through which the hairs protrude. These hairs are easily extracted on account of the inflammation at their root, which itself appears swollen. From the indurated mass pus oozes, which dries and forms thin yellow scabs, and when the eruption disappears cicatrices are left and the place remains bald. The disease is specially liable to follow attacks of eczema.

Diagnosis.—A. sycosis may be mistaken for A. vulgaris, eczema, or a syphilide. From them it may be distinguished because it always attacks the hairy parts alone, and does not spread beyond them, because the hairs pierce the pustules or tubercles, and no similar eruptions are seen elsewhere.

Prognosis.—The course is always tedious and the disease is difficult to cure, but it rarely terminates fatally unless erysipelas occurs as well.

Morbid Anatomy.—This is very much the same as in A. indurata, but differs in the greater length of the hair and their follicles and in the greater depth to which they penetrate the corium. The purulent foci, therefore, lie at a greater distance from the surface, and excite more severe inflammatory exudation into and hypertrophy of the tissues surrounding the follicles. Pus is also found outside the follicles and sebaceous glands and at the roots of the hairs, which are thus more or less completely destroyed. There is, however, no obstructing plug of sebum acting as a mechanical irritant, as in A. vulgaris.

Treatment.—This consists, in the first place, in epilating the hairs of the diseased parts and in shaving the rest of the patch, but to be of real service epilation should be commenced as early as possible in the attack and should be continued as it spreads. The pustules should be pricked and the pus let out, and if the part is not very painful or inflamed they should be lightly touched with acid nitrate of mercury, but if it is tender cold-water rags covered with oil silk should be applied. As the disease becomes more chronic ointments and lotions similar to those recommended in A. vulgaris should be tried. Hebra strongly insists on the importance of regular shaving after the disease has been cured, to prevent its recurrence.

ACNE ROSACEA.

Definition.—A disease of the skin occurring on the face, and characterised by great hyperæmia of the part and dilatation of the vessels, accompanied by hypertrophy of the fibrous elements and of the glands, which sometimes leads to the production of tumours.

Symptoms.—A. rosacea is believed to be to some extent hereditary, and is certainly due to some condition affecting the general health. Indigestion, produced by excess of food or strong drinks, causes flushing of the face, which often terminates in this disease, and in women irregularities of menstruation must also be mentioned. It may appear at any time except during childhood, but generally in middle or advanced life.

A. rosacea is not in itself a disease of the sebaceous glands, although they are frequently among the tissues affected. It is always limited to the face, and attacks in preference the nose, cheeks, forehead, and chin. It commences by an injection of the blood vessels, leading to a reddening of the skin, which fades on pressure and is increased greatly after a meal or on exposure to cold. This hyperæmia of the part produces a burning or tingling sensation. The disease may stop at this stage or may be associated with other morbid changes, but when these are absent the nose is usually alone affected. With the reddening there may be a considerable increase in the amount of sebum secreted, which gives the part a very greasy appearance, or the sebaceous glands may be inflamed and filled with secretion and their ducts remain open. At a later stage round nodules form, and great hypertrophy of the part takes place, which, when the nose is attacked, causes great deformity. The nodules may be of varying shape and size, and sometimes hang from the nose in pendulous masses.

The disease may persist or the redness may fade, and the tubercles either become absorbed or drop off, but extensive suppuration and ulceration never occurs.

Diagnosis.—A. rosacea has to be distinguished from A. vulgaris, lupus erythematosus, and on the nose from frost-bite.

From the first it may be recognised by the limitation of A. rosacea to the face, while A. vulgaris attacks the chest and back, and also because the inflammation in the former affects the skin between the acne spots and causes a tingling sensation.

From lupus erythematosus A. rosacea can be distinguished by the absence of ulceration and of the scabs which are present in the former.

From frost-bite the early stage of A. rosacea is also distinguished by the amount of swelling, and the dark purple, shining appearance in frost-bite contrasts with the bright red and greasy appearance in A. rosacea.

Prognosis.—It is never fatal, but is very obstinate, lasting sometimes for life.

Morbid Anatomy.—The anatomy of A. rosacea cannot be clearly described, but there is no doubt that the disease begins with hyperæmia of the part and increased growth of the fibrous and connective tissue, and that hypertrophy of the glands also takes place.

Treatment.—Regulation of the diet and, when necessary, of the menses, should be attended to before any good result can be expected from local treatment. The inunction of sulphur or iodide of sulphur ointment, the application of a weak solution of perchloride of mercury, or lightly touching the spots with acid nitrate of mercury, are the best forms of local treatment, but three or four days must frequently be allowed to intervene in order that the inflammation excited by this treatment may have time to subside.

In the more severe form the local hyperæmia is relieved by frequent multiple linear scarifications, and when any great deformity exists the complete removal of the tubercular excrescence is desirable.

MOLLUSCUM CONTAGIOSUM.

Definition.—A contagious disease of the skin, affecting the sebaceous glands, leading to the blocking up of the duct and an increased growth of the gland, which becomes filled with a white fatty and granular substance.

Symptoms.—The cause of the disease is unknown, but there is no doubt that it can be communicated from one person to another, although the mode has not been yet discovered. The disease appears first as a minute hard, white, shiny swelling, which gradually grows until it becomes as large as a hazel nut, but it is usually about the size of a pea. This little tumour, which may be sessile or pedunculated, is circular in form, with a flat top, having in its centre a small depression, which is the mouth of a sebaceous gland, and from which, when the tumour is squeezed, a soft, white, milky substance is forced. The tumours may occur singly or in scattered groups on the face, especially the eyelids, chest, arms, genitals, and on the breasts in women, and cause no pain, tenderness, or irritation, but occasionally producing, when inflamed, an ecthymatous pustule. As the tumours dry up small horns or warts are sometimes left. The disease is more common in children than in adults.

Diagnosis.—It is easily recognised by the umbilication and ease with which the tumour can be emptied, and is not liable to be mistaken for any other disease.

Morbid Anatomy.—The white material of which the tumour is composed is found to consist of granular and fatty matter with altered epithelium cells. On examining vertical sections some of the tumours are seen to be composed of cystlike dilatations of sebaceous glands filled with the products of the broken-down epithelial lining. Others present a lobulated structure, and microscopically are seen to be enclosed in fibrous capsules, which send delicate septa between the lobules. In each lobule there is first a layer of columnar cells next the fibrous wall, and then two or three layers of polygonal cells more or less infiltrated with fat globules, whilst the centre is occupied by roundish or oval bodies, the so-called 'molluscum corpuscles,' mixed with some fatty débris. These oval bodies, which were formerly supposed to be peculiar to molluscum, are merely epithelial cells that have undergone lardaceous or albuminoid degeneration.

The whole tumour is covered by the superficial portion of the corium, which is somewhat thinned and has its papillæ flattened by the pressure of the subjacent growth. Its walls and base are surrounded by a network of fine vessels, which bleed when the tumour is snipped off.

Treatment.—Treatment consists in making an incision across the tumour with a sharp knife and then squeezing out the contents.

SUBDIVISION B.—Of the Sweat Glands.

HYPERIDROSIS.

Definition.—A condition characterised by excessive sweating, which may be general or local.

Symptoms.—General sweating may occur in the course of any of the acute constitutional diseases, such as acute rheumatism, when the whole surface of the body may be bathed in perspiration.

Local sweating may affect the hands or feet, or one hand or foot, or even one-half of the body, and produces a sodden appearance, such as is seen after prolonged immersion in water. From the constant irritation of the sweat eczema may result.

Treatment.—This should depend on the cause, internal remedies, such as belladonna, being required if the sweating is general. Sponging with vinegar and water is useful to check the night sweats in phthisis. Locally the part should be constantly washed with yellow soap and water, and bathed with a lead or tannic acid lotion.

ANIDROSIS.

Definition.—A condition characterised by a deficiency of perspiration, and occurring as a result either of a constitutional disease or of an altered state of the skin, as in ichthyosis.

BROMIDROSIS.

Definition.—A condition characterised by the odour of the perspiration.

Symptoms.—This disease may be general or local. The former occurs usually in the course of some constitutional disease, when the smell differs according to the variety. Local bromidrosis is normally present in certain regions of the body, such as the axillæ, perineum, and feet, and it can therefore only be considered a disease when the smell is excessive. When the feet are affected the odour is at times so offensive that the person is unable to attend to his duties, though his general health is perfectly good. The perspiration is greatly increased above the normal, and is quickly absorbed by the socks, from which the smell arises, owing to rapid decomposition.

Treatment.—Local bromidrosis is often very difficult to cure. Thorough cleanliness is essential; the part should be washed at least twice daily with plenty of soap, then dried and powdered with starch or flour. Sea-water baths at night are of value in some cases, and so also is painting the whole part occasionally with iodine. In severe cases, when other measures fail, Hebra recommends the following plan, which he says 'will invariably be attended with success':—

'A certain quantity of the simple diachylon plaister (emp. plumbi, emp. lithargyri) is to be melted over a gentle fire, and an equal weight of linseed oil is then to be incorporated with it, the product being stirred till a homogeneous mass is produced, sufficiently adhesive not to crumble readily to pieces. This is then to be spread over a piece of linen measuring about a square foot. The foot of the patient, having been first well washed and thoroughly dried, is now to be wrapped in the dressing thus prepared. Pledgets of lint on which the same ointment has been spread are also to be introduced into the space between each pair of toes, to prevent their touching one another; and care must be taken that the foot is completely covered, and that the dressing is accurately in contact with the skin. When this has been done an ordinary sock or stocking may be put on the foot, and outside this a new shoe, which must be light and should not cover the dorsum of the foot. After twelve hours the dressing is to be removed; the foot is then not to be washed, but must be rubbed with a dry cloth. The dressing is then to be renewed in the same way as before, and its application is afterwards to be repeated twice a day. This procedure must be continued for eight to twelve days, according to the severity of the case. . . . In the course of a few days it will be found that a brownish-yellow cuticle, about $\frac{1}{2}'''$ thick, is be ginning to peel off from all those parts of the skin which were before affected with the disease, and that a healthy, clean, white surface of epidermis is exposed as this substance separates.'

CHROMIDROSIS.

Definition.—A very rare condition in which the sweat is said to be coloured.

SUDAMINA—MILIARIA.

Definition.—An eruption of small transparent vesicles, chiefly on the abdomen, which contain sweat.

Symptoms.—In the course of an acute disease, in which excessive sweating is a prominent feature, small transparent vesicles suddenly appear. At first sight they look like drops of water on the surface, but they are hard to touch. The vesicles contain sweat, which is proved by analysis. When they burst an eczema may result from the irritation of the sweat.

Treatment.—None is required, unless the disease is accompanied by eczema, which should be treated accordingly.

CHAPTER XXII.

SUBDIVISION C.—*Of the Hair.*

Hirsuties—Lichen pilaris—Nævus pilosus—Canities—Alopecia—
Alopecia areata—Trichorexis nodosa.

SUBDIVISION D.—*Of the Nails.*

Onychia—Onychogryphosis—Onychauxis— Onychatrophia—In
General Diseases.

SUBDIVISION C.—*Of the Hair.*

HIRSUTIES.

HIRSUTIES, or an excessive growth of hair on parts where normally only fine down occurs, may be either congenital or acquired.

In the congenital variety the excessive growth may be either diffuse, covering the whole surface or a large portion of it, as in the so-called 'hairy men,' or localised to certain smaller areæ, as in moles or nævi.

In the acquired variety large hairs, more or less numerous, develope in places generally covered only with lanuginous hairs, such as the upper lip or chin of women, the areola of the nipple, or on warts. The irritation of the skin by blisters or stimulating applications produces in some individuals an abundant growth of long downy or bristly hairs.

The process consists usually of an increase in number and a closer aggregation of the hairs, which are occasionally thick and bristly. The condition does not affect the general health, and is only troublesome in consequence of the disfigurement it produces.

Treatment.—When the hairs are scanty and long, epilation is the best mode of removing them; but when they are numerous, and are situated on the lip or chin of women, a depilatory paste, containing orpiment and slaked lime or sulphide of calcium, may be applied every three or four days.

LICHEN PILARIS.

Lichen pilaris consists in the development of small papular swellings around the hair follicles, and affects the extensor surfaces of the limbs. On the outer side of the thighs, where they are most frequently observed, the skin feels rough and harsh to the touch. The papules, which are about the size of a pin's head, are pale, or only slightly hyperæmic, and do not itch or cause any other subjective sensation.

Morbid Anatomy.—The papules are due to epithelial débris accumulating in and blocking up the mouth of a hair follicle, with usually some exudation into and hypertrophy of the connective tissue around the neck of the follicle.

Treatment.—This consists in washing the skin thoroughly with soap and water, frequent warm baths, and in the inunction of vaseline or some simple ointment.

NÆVUS PILOSUS—HAIRY MOLE.

Nævus pilosus is the term applied to the brown pigmented patches, covered usually with long hairs, which are usually congenital.

They are smooth and level with the surface, or only slightly raised, and consist of slight hypertrophy of the papillary layer, in which and in the rete much brown or black pigment is deposited, while the hairs are considerably hypertrophied. The patches are sometimes the starting points of melanotic sarcomatous growths.

Treatment.—They can be destroyed by blistering or with potassa fusa or other caustics, or by scraping with Volkmann's spoon.

CANITIES.

Canities is the term applied to the blanching of the hair, occurring normally as a gradual senile change or suddenly under the influence of severe mental emotions. The change begins at the root of the hair by a diminished formation of pigment, and a papilla which has once produced a grey hair does not usually form coloured ones. The sudden alteration is ascribed to a development of air bubbles in the substance of the hair shaft, which obscure the pigment present in the medullary portion. Sometimes canities occurs as a result of disease of the hair follicles, but after a time the hairs may become recoloured.

ALOPECIA—BALDNESS.

Deficient growth of hair may be either congenital or acquired. The former is rare, and in it the hair is scanty and downy, or entirely absent from the scalp, but usually after a time the growth may become normal. Acquired baldness may result either as a senile change, when it is often preceded by greyness of the hair with more or less atrophy of the skin, sebaceous glands, and hair follicles, or at a comparatively early period as a sequel of one of the acute diseases, such as scarlatina, erysipelas, &c., or as a result of a local inflammatory process which affects the hair follicles and papillæ, as in acute or chronic eczema, psoriasis, syphilis, favus, ringworm, &c.

In *alopecia senilis* the skin, hair follicles, and glands are diminished in size and wasted, and only fine lanuginous hairs are produced. The change is a permanent one and not amenable to treatment.

In *premature alopecia*, resulting from acute diseases, the baldness is usually temporary. In eczema, psoriasis, and other affections the shedding of the hair is analogous to the desquamation of the cuticle from the inflamed skin, and, unless the inflammation has been sufficiently severe to destroy the hair papillæ, new hair, at first downy and afterwards normal, is reproduced. But where the follicles and the papillæ have been destroyed by suppuration and ulceration the baldness is permanent, and no treatment is of any avail. For the loss of hair after fevers tonics, generous diet, and a local stimulating lotion containing cantharides are the proper measures to be relied upon.

ALOPECIA AREATA.

Definition.—An atrophic disease characterised by the sudden loss of hair in small roundish limited patches, which have a tendency to enlarge slowly.

Symptoms.—The disease begins on the head or beard by the sudden loss of hair on a limited area. The hair comes out easily, and shows no sign of brittleness or any morbid change. Usually there is no sensation to indicate the position of the disease. The patches from which the hair has fallen are extremely smooth, white, and glistening, or polished like a billiard ball, and on the same level with or slightly more depressed than the adjacent skin. The patches are most common on the scalp, but may occur on the eyebrows, cheeks, or other hairy parts of the body; they are sharply limited and surrounded by healthy hair, growing luxuriantly.. As the disease spreads the hairs at the margin of the patch become loose and easily fall out, and thus by the confluence of patches large irregular areæ are formed. After a time the disease becomes spontaneously arrested, the smooth shiny skin becomes marked by little prominences corresponding to the hair follicles, and thin hairs, at first white and downy, but afterwards stronger and darker, are slowly reproduced. In rare instances the hair never grows again, or only as fine, pale, downy threads.

Diagnosis.—The patches of alopecia areata are sometimes mistaken for tinea tonsurans, but the differences between the two diseases are so marked that the diagnosis is easy. In tinea tonsurans the patches are rarely bald, but are covered with short stubby hair, which comes out easily and under the microscope shows the fungoid character of the disease. The patches are also scaly, contrasting strongly with the perfectly smooth, shiny patches of alopecia areata.

Prognosis.—The disease, arising suddenly, like zoster and morphœa, runs a definite though prolonged course, and tends to spontaneous recovery. It is probably a neurosis, and due to some nutritive lesion affecting the formation and growth of the hair. The occasional occurrence of alopecia areata on neuralgic patches is a fact somewhat in favour of this view.

Morbid Anatomy.—No visible changes have been discovered in the cutis. The bulbs of the affected hairs are atrophied, and a nodular swelling, due to the inversion of the root sheath on them, is sometimes seen near the end. The fungus described by Gruby, Bazin, and some others, and named micosporon Audoninii, has not been found by the majority of modern observers, and the cases described as alopecia areata by the first-named observers were probably only old-standing and severe forms of ringworm in which the hair had been completely destroyed. Inoculations from true alopecia areata have not produced any result (Dyce Duckworth).

Treatment.—The spreading of the disease can sometimes be arrested, and the new growth of hair encouraged, by severe blistering with acetum cantharidis or Burt's vesicating fluid. The blistering should be repeated every fortnight. Internally iron, strychnine, arsenic, and other nervine tonics are said to be of value; at all events they should be tried in conjunction with local stimulation.

TRICHOREXIS NODOSA.

Trichorexis nodosa consists in the formation of little oval or round swellings on the hairs of the beard and moustache. The little nodes look like nits, but are seen under the microscope to be formed by a localised splitting and bulging of the hair itself, which presents somewhat the appearance of two brooms thrust into one another. No parasite is present, and the condition is ascribed by Beigel, who first described it, to the generation of gas in the medulla bursting the cortical substance of the hair. The affected hairs are not more easily extracted than normal hairs, but they break very readily at the nodes, leaving a frayed, brushlike extremity. The disease is very common and of little consequence. The treatment usually recommended is shaving, though the hairs are apt to split again when allowed to grow.

SUBDIVISION D.—*Of the Nails.*

ONYCHIA.

Inflammation of the nails occurs after mechanical injuries to the matrix, such, for instance, as pressure on the edges of an hypertrophied toe nail (paronychia lateralis), or spontaneously after a slight scratch or tear of the skin about the fold round the nail.

There is redness and swelling of the fold round the nail, most marked at the sides near each angle in 'ingrowing toe nail,' together with a deep red discoloration of the matrix, attended with great tenderness on pressure and a sensation of heat and throbbing. The nail on its margin in idiopathic onychia becomes opaque, pus collects under it and under the cuticle of the fold, and the nail, becoming loosened in places, covers a sloughy, raw, tender surface, from which a brownish-red fluid exudes. Frequently the whole nail is shed, and after a slow process of healing a new nail forms, which is thin, rough, and brittle. In 'ingrowing toe nail' the inflammation and subsequent suppuration is limited to one or other angle of the nail and to the adjacent nail fold, from which exuberant tender granulations protrude.

In acute onychia, or 'whitlow,' there is often pyrexia and constitutional disturbance, and necrosis of the terminal phalanx, suppuration in the synovial sheaths, and cellulitis of the hand and arm may occur.

Treatment.—'Ingrowing toe nail' in its milder forms may be well treated, as suggested by Dr. Tilbury Fox, by scraping the centre of the nail quite thin with a piece of glass and softening

s

it with liquor potassæ. The granulations should be touched
with nitrate of silver from time to time. Should the disease be
more advanced, the nail should be completely removed by operation. In acute onychia, or 'whitlow,' poultices should be applied to the part, to promote suppuration ; dead skin or nail must
be removed, and subsequently it should be dressed with astringent lotions. Internally tonics and stimulants should be prescribed.

ONYCHOGRYPHOSIS.

This is the term applied to a condition observed most frequently in the little and great toes, in which the central portion
of the nail becomes converted into an irregular clawlike or horny
growth, ridged and more opaque and brittle than the normal
nail. It is due to the local hypertrophy of the papillæ of the
matrix and of the nail bed in front of it, as a result of continued
pressure.

The papillæ, sometimes two or three lines in length, project
into the horny mass and form a tender, vascular core embedded
in greatly thickened epithelial layers, as seen in ichthyosis.

ONYCHAUXIS.

Onychauxis, or hypertrophy of the nail, assumes either the
form of a lateral outgrowth which may press upon and irritate
the adjacent folds of skin, causing the so-called 'ingrowing toe
nail,' or in the form of a somewhat chisel-shaped thickening of
the nail, with the thick, broad part at the free border produced by
hypertrophy of the papillæ in the anterior part of the nail bed.

The condition is analogous to tyloma, as onychogryphosis
is to clavus.

Treatment.—Both these forms of undue growth of nail substance can be treated by paring away the excess of horny substance by means of the knife, scissors, or pliers. Should the
soft, vascular part be exposed, it should be divided and the
bleeding spot rapidly cauterised.

ONYCHATROPHIA.

Absence or defective development of the nails occurs some-- times as a congenital condition, and frequently in association with absence of hair. The more common variety results from disease or destruction of the matrix or bed of the nail in the course of various local or general diseases, but most usually from injury.

IN GENERAL DISEASES.

The changes met with in the nails as a result of general or local disease may be classed under the following heads :—

1. *Acute.*—Desquamative, in erysipelas, scarlatina, pity- riasis rubra, and acute eczema.
2. *Chronic.*—From severe diseases, such as enteric fever, pneumonia, peritonitis, &c.
3. In chronic eczema, psoriasis, and lichen ruber.
4. As a result of parasitic growths in favus and tinea cir- cinata.

1. In acute eczema, erysipelas, scarlatina, and pityriasis rubra, the nails are sometimes shed as a consequence of the local hyperæmia and exudation, the process being of the same nature as the desquamation of the cuticle.

2. After severe diseases, such as enteric fever, pneumonia, and acute rheumatism, depressed transverse lines are often found on the nails during convalescence. The nail at these places is much thinner than normal, and often somewhat opaque and brittle.

3. In chronic eczema, when the disease attacks the hands or feet, it may spread to the nails, causing them at first to become pitted like the rind of an orange. Later they split longitudi- nally, at first slightly, when the dirt which fills the cracks makes them look like black lines, but widening as the disease progresses until the whole nail splits from end to end and finally is shed.

s 2

In psoriasis the nails may become thickened, opaque, irregular, and darker in colour. They are very brittle, short, fissured at their extremities, and present transverse cracks. In the bed and under the margin small spots of psoriasis may be seen in the early stages of the disease.

In lichen ruber, in severe cases, the nails are opaque, rough, and brittle, sometimes thickened, and at others times thin and atrophied.

4. In some cases of tinea tonsurans and of favus the nails become affected with the fungus growth. They are irregular, thickened, and brittle, and in places are marked with yellowish spots and lines, in which the nail is more friable than normal and appears rotten. Under the microscope, after soaking in liquor potassæ, scrapings show mycelium filaments and the spores of trichophyton or achorion.

CHAPTER XXIII.

Class A.—PARASITIC AFFECTIONS.

Sub-class A.—*Animal.*

Pediculosis—Scabies—Eruptions produced by Fleas, Bugs, &c.

Sub-class B.—*Vegetable.*

Tinea tonsurans—Kerion—Tinea sycosis—Tinea circinata—Eczema marginatum—Tinea versicolor—Tinea favosa.

Sub-class A.—*Animal.*

PEDICULOSIS—PHTHIRIASIS.

Definition.—A diseased condition of the skin produced by the attacks of lice.

Symptoms.—Three species of lice infest the human body—*pediculus capitis*, restricted to the hairy scalp; *pediculus pubis*, found about the genitals, and occasionally on the margins of the eyelids, beard, and axillæ; and *pediculus corporis*, or vestimenti, chiefly affecting the trunk.

In *pediculosis capitis*, produced by the presence of pediculi capitis, the lice are found wandering about the roots of the hair, most abundantly on the occipital and temporal regions, and more frequently in women and children than in male adults. They excite intense itching by thrusting their probosces into the hair follicles and sucking blood from the capillaries, and soon, owing to the scratching which results, excoriations, eczematous eruptions, and crusts appear. The hair becomes matted, foul-smelling, and covered with adherent 'nits' or ova; the glands in the anterior triangle and at the back of the neck frequently swell and even suppurate, and excoriated spots and boils often appear on the nape of the neck.

In *pediculosis pubis*, the *crab lice*, as they are termed from their shape, anchor themselves firmly to the roots of the pubic hairs, and by their sucking produce itching and follicular irritation, which excites scratching and thereby causes excoriations and eczema. The lice are seen as little greyish specks adhering to the bases of the hairs, and are mostly found in adults.

Pediculosis corporis, occurring mostly in elderly persons, like the previous affection, is excited by lice, which, however, are rarely visible on stripping the patient, as they inhabit and deposit their ova in the folds of the under-clothing and the interstices of flannel garments worn next the skin. Thrusting their proboscis into the hair follicles, they wound the capillaries and produce minute hæmorrhagic specks, surrounded at first, like flea-bites, by a hyperæmic zone. These spots are the seats of intense itching or creeping sensations. Violent scratching ensues; the cuticle is torn off over the parts affected, and excoriations are produced, covered by scabs of dried blood. Papular, urticarial, eczematous, and furuncular or pustular eruptions are usually excited in the same way, and in old-standing cases the skin becomes deeply pigmented and covered with scabs, which are most numerous about the shoulders and the front of the chest beneath the clavicles. This eruption was formerly named prurigo senilis, and is not pathognomonic of pediculi in itself, being capable of production by any intense itching, but its restriction to certain sites and the presence of hæmorrhagic puncta determine the diagnosis.

Diagnosis.—In *pediculosis capitis* the presence of the 'nits' or ova— small whitish, semi-translucent bodies—firmly adherent to the hairs, and the discovery of the parasites near their roots or attaching to the comb, settles the question.

In *pediculosis pubis* the parasites adhere to the roots of the hairs, and have the appearance of little greyish or brownish scales, which when pulled off with forceps often tear out the hair to which they cling.

In *pediculosis corporis* the lice must be looked for on the folds of the under-clothing, about the junctions of the sleeves with the body, and under the collar of the shirt. The restriction of the 'pruritic rash' to the shoulders and infraclavicular region, and the presence of hæmorrhagic puncta, may occasionally, when, from the under-clothing having recently been changed, no pediculi can be found thereon, lead to an accurate diagnosis.

Prognosis.—Pediculi, if untreated, may increase and multiply for years, causing eczema, pruritic eruptions, glandular enlargements, abscesses, &c. Under appropriate measures, however, they are readily exterminated, and the eruptions excited by them subside either spontaneously or under ordinary treatment in a short time.

Anatomy.—The pediculus belongs to the class Insecta. Its head, which is small, is furnished with a delicate retractile proboscis, not usually discernible after death; and it has a compressed thorax, six legs, and a somewhat flattened abdomen.

The pediculus capitis has a slender shape, and is generally smaller than the other varieties; its abdomen is ovoid and terminates in a blunt cone.

The pediculus corporis is much larger, averaging $\frac{1}{14}$ to $\frac{1}{8}$ inch in length; its abdomen presents a terminal triangular notch.

The pediculus pubis, the crab louse, is relatively much broader and shorter than the other kinds; its abdomen is nodulated, and the anterior pairs of its short stout legs are provided with strong claws, with which it anchors itself firmly to the skin.

Treatment.—The full-grown lice are easily destroyed by a carbolic lotion (1 to 20), or by the inunction of dilute ammonio-chloride, red precipitate ointment, oleate of mercury 5 per cent., or ung. hyd. c. sulph. As the ova are not readily attacked by these remedies, they must be applied for a week or ten days, so as to destroy the young lice as they become hatched.

For pediculus pubis, ung. staphisagriæ, scented with oil of lavender or roses, is a very valuable application.

Pediculus corporis should be treated by warm baths, thorough change of clothing, and baking the old garments in a disinfecting oven at a temperature of 250°–300° Fahr., so as to destroy the lice or their ova.

Itching may be mitigated by soothing alkaline or prussic acid and glycerine lotions, and any eczematous or other eruptions treated on general principles.

SCABIES—ITCH.

Definition.—A contagious disease of the skin, produced by the presence of the acarus scabiei in the epidermis.

Symptoms.—Following the arrangement of Hebra, we may class the phenomena of scabies under three headings, viz.—

1. Those arising directly from the presence of acari in the skin.
2. Those which are the result of scratching.
3. Those which are produced by the action of other irritants upon portions of skin affected by acari.

1. Those directly due to the presence of acari in the skin.

The full-grown female acarus after impregnation begins at once to work her way into the epidermis, and burrows somewhat obliquely under the surface into the soft cells of the stratum lucidum or the rete, giving rise to a narrow, somewhat sinuous tunnel or cuniculus. The tunnel, whitish, and dotted here and there with darkish spots—six or eight in number, which are the deposited ova—is somewhat dilated at its terminal extremity into a small roundish chamber, in which the acarus lies. At times the burrow is seen as a whitish line on the summit of a reddish ridge, and occasionally vesicles or pustules form near to or along the course of the cuniculus, but never involve its terminal chamber. At the extremities the burrows, which average $\frac{1}{5}$th of an inch in length, but which may vary from $\frac{1}{25}$th of an inch to two or three inches, are usually blackened by contact with staining materials, dirt, &c., on the trunk, penis, buttocks, elbows, and knees, and in the skin of children; while upon the hands of very cleanly people they are pale and not easily detected. In adults the disease most frequently attacks the inter-digital webs and the thin skin on the flexor surface of the wrist ; it also attacks the penis, hypogastrium, the buttocks, axillæ or flexures of the elbows, mammæ, and inner ankles. In children the buttocks and feet are the chief seats of the disease, but any part of the body may become inoculated. The scalp and face are never implicated in adults, and only very rarely in children. The burrowing of the acarus is accompanied by itching, which is worst at night; and by the irritation of the parasite alone, as well as by the scratching it excites, urticarial, eczematous, pustular, or ecthymatous eruptions may be produced.

2. As a result of scratching linear wheals, excoriated papules covered with black crusts of dried blood, vesicles, pustules, &c., are usually developed, forming a ' pruritic rash ' similar to that of pediculosis. It is always most marked on the front of the trunk and thighs, being limited to, or at all events. most intense on, a space bounded by the mammary line above and the knees below. The face is very seldom scratched, and the back to a less extent than the front of the trunk.

3. If the skin affected with itch be exposed to pressure or friction, papules, tubercles, pustules, or crusts appear over the tubera ischii—e.g. when persons sit on hard benches—or they. may present themselves on the tracts of skin indurated by crutches, trusses, belts, garters, or tight clothes. These nodules may or may not exhibit burrows on their summits.

Diagnosis.—The diagnosis of scabies is based upon the history of contagion, usually to be elicited, the steady progress of the affection, the presence of itching, aggravated at night, the particular site of the eruption, on the wrists and between the fingers most frequently in adults (unless parasiticide soaps be used), on the penis, hypogastrium, and mammæ, or on the buttocks and feet, in infants, and by the discovery of cuniculi, from the terminal dilatations of which the acari can be extracted and examined microscopically.

When, as in infants, the burrows cannot be easily distinguished and crusts are abundant, the maceration of these with liquor potassæ will often assist the discovery of full-grown or embryonic acari.

Attention to these distinctive features will simplify the diagnosis of scabies, even though it should be complicated with pruritic, eczematous, or ecthymatous eruptions.   Prurigo of Hebra differs from scabies by the presence of hard, solid, fleshy papules, by its history, and by the greater severity of the itching.

In pediculosis corporis, as in scabies, a ' pruritic rash ' may be present upon the trunk, but the absence of cuniculi in the skin will sufficiently distinguish the former from the latter.

Prognosis.—Scabies is merely a local trouble ; exerts no deteriorating influence on the constitution even in inveterate cases. It usually yields to parasiticides, and the eczematous eruptions excited by it and by the scratching subside under suitable treatment.

Anatomy.—The adult female acarus scabiei is oval, about $\frac{1}{80}$th to $\frac{1}{60}$th of an inch long by $\frac{1}{100}$th to $\frac{1}{80}$th of an inch broad ; the dorsal surface is convex and armed with angular spines, while the ventral presents four pairs of legs, the two anterior of which have stalked suckers.   In the male the third pair are furnished with fine setæ, and the fourth with suckers.   In the female both hinder pairs are provided with setæ only, and, whereas the male wanders upon the surface, she burrows into the cuticle and deposits from twelve to twenty ova, from which are hatched six-legged embryos.   These undergo several changes of skin, and acquire their fourth pair of legs after the first moulting.

Treatment.—Give a warm bath, wash well with soap, thoroughly rub in some parasiticide ointment, containing as the essential ingredient grs. xx to ʒss of sulphur to ʒj of lard, scented with various aromatic oils ; put on close-fitting flannel drawers and jerseys, so as to keep the ointment acting upon the skin ; and repeat the bath and the washing at the end of forty-eight hours.   If itching continues after this, the same plan must be adopted again.   Care must be taken not to use too strong preparations of sulphur, as they are apt to produce a severe ecze-matous condition. As a substitute balsam of Peru, or storax in the form of an ointment, may be tried. Sulphur vapour baths have been recommended, but they are not so efficacious as the other modes of treatment.

ERUPTIONS PRODUCED BY FLEAS, BUGS, ETC.

The common flea, *pulex irritans*, gives rise to a roseolar spot, sometimes slightly raised, with a central red punctum, and as the redness fades the centre remains as a red or dark-coloured petechia, lasting several days, and known as the purpura pulicosa. In some persons urticarial wheals or vesicles may result.

The bed bug, *acanthia lectularia*, causes erythematous or urticarial spots, which itch much and are more persistent than flea bites. Though the redness fades in a day or so, a small itchy, indurated papule with central hæmorrhagic punc-tum may last two or three days more.

The harvest mite, *leptus autumnalis*, a minute reddish para-site, belonging, like the itch insect, to the class Arachnida, embeds itself in the skin, and causes a papular eruption with itching, intensified at night as the temperature of the body increases. The appearance lasts a week or ten days and then subsides.

Gnats and mosquitoes, belonging to the genus Culex, and some kinds of midges also, cause erythematous or urticarial papules, and similar eruptions, which itch intensely, are excited in some persons by the hairs of a certain class of caterpillars.

Treatment.—The itching may be allayed by the applica-tion of diluted sp. amm. aromat., of lot. carbonis detergens (ʒj to ℥j), or lot. hydrarg. perchlor. grs. ij to ℥j with the addition of ℞x to ℞xii of dilute prussic acid in the ounce.

Sub-class B.—*Vegetable*.

Some authors, among them Hebra and Neumann, are of opinion that all skin diseases caused by the growth of fungi in the epidermis or appendages are due to one species of parasite, which presents certain differences according to the conditions of the nidus in which it is found. It is more usual, however, to describe three different varieties of fungi, viz.—

   a. Trichophyton tonsurans.
   b. Microsporon furfur.
   c. Achorion Schoenleinii.

Trichophyton tonsurans, occurring in various parts of the body, gives rise to cutaneous affections, to which the term tinea with some qualifying adjective has usually been applied. In the scalp it causes *tinea tonsurans*, the common ringworm, and *kerion* where prominent, boggy, honey-combed patches are present. On the hairy parts of the face it produces *tinea sycosis*, on the body *tinea circinata* (herpes circinatus, &c.), and the so-called *eczema marginatum*. The nails also occasionally become affected. The disease attacks all classes, the healthy and prosperous as well as the poor and debilitated.

TINEA TONSURANS—RINGWORM OF THE HEAD.

Definition.—A contagious disease of the scalp, cau.ed by the presence of trichophyton tonsurans in the epidermis, the hairs and their follicles.

Symptoms.—Tinea tonsurans is met with most frequently in children, but is occasionally seen in adults. From the fact that persons who have suffered long from ringworm of the scalp in childhood frequently present patches of tinea versicolor when grown up, it has been supposed that the latter affection is due to a modification of the trichophyton, produced by the difference between the skin of an adult and that of a child. In the early stage, which rarely comes under observation, a small red, erythematous or slightly raised patch arises on some part of the hairy scalp, accompanied by considerable itching. As the patch gradually enlarges the redness and elevation of the centre subside, and a roundish ring with a bright red raised margin, often presenting a crop of small vesicles (herpes circinatus), and a paler rough or scurfy-looking centre is produced. If the rings be concentric, an eruption simulating erythema or herpes iris is produced.

In the fully developed condition ringworm appears as a pale brown or slaty-looking, roundish patch ($\frac{1}{2}$ inch to 3 or 4 inches in diameter), slightly elevated above the adjacent healthy scalp, and covered with short stubbly hairs $\frac{1}{8}$ inch long and small opaque branny scales. The hairs are thick, twisted, or bent, frayed at their extremities, have a dull greyish look, and break off or fall out easily from their follicles, which are somewhat prominent. At this stage the brittleness, loss of colour, and deformity of the stubbly hairs are marked features, and should always be looked for. In some instances the parasite excites an acute inflammation of the hair follicles, which become pustular, and as a consequence destruction of the papillæ of the hairs and permanent alopecia may follow.

Eczema is sometimes produced, and the yellowish-green, brittle crusts which then form conceal the appearances of ringworm.

Occasionally ringworm of the scalp becomes *diffuse*, and much resembles eczema capitis in the scaly stage. After lasting for a variable time ringworm begins to subside, and the patch is covered with fine scales and young hairs, which are apparently normal; or both skin and hairs may, on superficial observation, appear quite natural. Here and there, however, and chiefly at the margins of the patch, short, stubbly, discoloured hairs can be found on careful examination, and unless these are eradicated the disease is liable to relapse and to affect other persons.

In a few cases smooth, hairless patches, resembling those of alopecia areata, are produced, which, according to Dr. Liveing, has led to the erroneous belief that there is a parasitic disease (which has been called *tinea decalvans*) distinct, on the one hand, from tinea tonsurans, and on the other from alopecia areata.

KERION.

This is a rare condition, in which one or more of the patches of ordinary ringworm becomes raised, tender, and uneven; small prominences, resembling inflamed hair follicles, soon appear, from which a viscid, honeylike secretion exudes, and the whole mass becomes what may be termed ' boggy ' to the touch. As a rule no pus is formed, but the hairs and their follicles are gradually destroyed, the result being permanent baldness.

TINEA SYCOSIS.

This variation is produced when the parasite attacks the hair of the beard and moustache, and extends into their deep-seated follicles. The primary symptom, as in tinea tonsurans, is a red, scaly, and itching patch; the follicles next become indurated and tender, forming reddish, prominent tubercles, which suppurate; the hairs become dull and brittle, and are easily extracted. When the pustules and small abscesses round the follicles burst, crusting takes place, but to a less extent than in eczema of the face.

TINEA CIRCINATA.

This results from the development of trichophyton on the non-hairy parts of the body; it appears most commonly on the face, neck, and trunk, and may or may not be accompanied by patches of tinea tonsurans; it also shows itself on the hands and arms of those attending to cases of ringworm of the scalp. Small reddish, somewhat raised, circular patches, covered with branny scales, and usually presenting a ring of minute vesicles at their margins, make their appearance, and are commonly attended by marked itching. Fading in the centre, the patch gradually extends at the mar_ins, which are usually vesicular (hence the name herpes circinatus), and forms 'fairy rings,' like those of other fungi. By the coalescence of these rings irregular circinate or gyrate bands are produced, the rings ceasing to extend and overlap where they blend, as if the material for their further growth had been exhausted in spots already affected with the disease. T. circinata, when it reaches the scalp or hairy parts of the face, gives rise to T. tonsurans or T. sycosis, and is often found in isolated patches in persons affected with those diseases, or in those who have come in contact with them.

ECZEMA MARGINATUM,

Affecting the genitals, the inner sides of the thighs, and the buttocks, is merely a variety of tinea circinata occurring in parts where the abundant perspiration, warmth, and friction predispose the skin to inflammatory action. The red, elevated, and itching patches fade in the centre, leaving it deeply pigmented, and at the raised margins vesicles, pustules, excoriations, or crusts are met with. It spreads in the same way and presents the same fungus as T. circinata. In some cases the parasite may not be found, though the eczema which it has started persists.

Diagnosis.—In T. tonsurans the round, scaly, itching patches on the scalp, the dull, brittle, or stubbly hairs, which are easily pulled out, and the reddish, spreading margin, while the centre is pale, are features which are diagnostic of the disease. When impetiginous crusts hide the whole patch, when smooth, bald patches occur, when new hairs are growing and the disease is receding, or when it is in the early stage and appears as an erythematous or vesicular patch, ringworm may be mistaken for eczema of the scalp, alopecia areata, or erythema vesicans. When the entire scalp is affected, it is almost impossible to distinguish it from scaly eczema of the scalp. In all these cases, however, the detection of the parasite in the stubbly hairs, crusts, or scales, after maceration in liq. potassæ, will clear up the difficulty. The frequent occurrence of T. circinata on other parts of the body, or the detection of dull, brittle, broken off or distorted, easily extracted hairs, will also help the diagnosis.

Even to the naked eye the appearances of T. kerion are so peculiar that the nature of the affection can hardly be mistaken. In the early stages, where the puffy swelling may simulate a subcutaneous abscess, microscopical examination of the loosened hairs settles the question.

T. sycosis differs from eczema of the beard in the development of indurated tubercles and abscesses, the dull, brittle character of the hairs, which are readily extracted, the presence usually of T. circinata on other parts, and in the presence of trichophyton on microscopic examination. *T. circinata* and *eczema marginatum* may resemble some forms of erythema multiforme and of eczema respectively, but the spreading in 'fairy rings' and the presence of the parasite are diagnostic.

Prognosis.—Ringworm of the body is usually easily amenable to appropriate treatment, but on the hairy parts, on the other hand, it is extremely obstinate, persisting for months, and sometimes for years, in spite of all remedies, and being liable to recur if the treatment have been left off too soon. The parasite does not endanger life, but is troublesome on account of the loss of hair it causes, the secondary inflammations it sometimes excites, and the marked contagiousness of the affection.

Morbid Anatomy.—Examining under the microscope, after maceration for twenty-four hours in dilute liq. potassæ, the dull, brittle hairs or the epidermic scales obtained by scraping with a blunt knife a patch of tinea, fine mycelium filaments, made up of roundish or cylindrical segments, are seen running longitudinally throughout the hair, or forming a feltwork in and between the epidermic scales. Where the filaments reach the surface of the hair they give rise to globular aggregations (conidia), made up of minute round refracting bodies, the spores of the fungus, which measure about $\frac{1}{8000}$ inch in diameter. Occasionally no filaments are met with, the hair presenting only collections of conidia and scattered spores on the surface and in its substance.

Dr. F. Taylor, in examining vertical sections of a scalp affected with ringworm, found the following changes:—In hairs slightly affected mycelium filaments only were found, running along the length of the hair, which was not altered in shape. The hair was in later stages obscured by a dense aggregation of spores in its follicle, and its substance, as far down as the upper part of the bulb, was destroyed, or replaced by mycelium threads. The hair papillæ were never affected, and laterally the internal root-sheath formed the outer boundary of the fungus growth, no traces of it being found in the outer root-sheath, follicle walls, cutis, or epidermis. Only slight traces of inflammation were found round the hairs.

Treatment.—In the different varieties of tinea produced by trichophyton attention must be directed to—

1. The destruction of the parasite.

2. The removal of any secondary inflammation which may have been caused by the parasite or the remedies employed for its destruction.

Where the disease is superficial, as in T. circinata and eczema marginatum, there is little or no difficulty in carrying out the first indication. Lotions containing bichloride of mercury (grs. ij ad ʒj), sulphurous acid, or hyposulphite of soda (ʒj ad ʒj), or the persistent inunction of dilute ammonio-chloride or nitrate of mercury ointments, or of oleate of mercury 5 per cent., are usually curative in a few weeks. Vaseline, oleate of zinc, or bismuth, &c., should be used subsequently if there is any eczema.

In ringworm of the scalp or of the beard (T. sycosis) the main difficulty is to get the parasiticide brought into contact

T

with *all* the mycelial filaments and spores, many of which lie deep down in the hair follicles. Hence, though the superficial fungus growth is easily destroyed, and the disease appears to be eradicated, much annoyance is caused by the recurrence of the affection, a few conidia which have eluded the poison being sufficient to start a fresh growth, and subsequently to infect other persons.

The indications, therefore, for treatment are to—

1. Remove as much as possible of the diseased hairs and epidermis.

2. Use a parasiticide which will penetrate readily and deeply into the cuticle and hair follicles.

3. Continue the treatment, more or less modified, for at least a month after all signs of the disease are gone.

1. The hair over the diseased patch, and for $\frac{1}{4}$ to $\frac{1}{2}$ inch round, or of the whole scalp, beard, &c., should be cut short with scissors, all crusts removed by oiling or poulticing, and the surface washed well with soft soap and water. Loose hairs and scales should by removed by rubbing, and in the case of T. sycosis by epilation, which, owing to the loosening of the hairs, is here less painful than in eczema of the beard. Blistering by liq. epispasticus, acetum cantharidis glaciale, or Coster's paint of iodine and oil of wood tar, is also useful for this purpose.

2. A solution of bichloride of mercury in acetic acid (grs. vj to ʒiv), which has the combined advantages of penetrating deeply, of macerating the hair and epidermic tissues, and of blistering, is one of the best. It should be repeated from time to time, and weak acid nitrate or ammonio-chloride of mercury ointments applied in the intervals to the irritated skin.

3. After removing all the stubbly hairs, and when no further reproduction of the disease has appeared for some time after the last application of vesicants or of the mercury and acetic acid paint, weak ammonio-chloride of mercury ointment should be rubbed in twice a day for some time further, to guard against the possibility of some overlooked portion of fungus starting into fresh growth.

Any eczema of the scalp thus excited should be treated in the usual way.

Goa powder, or its active principle, chrysophanic acid, are useful only as irritants, and do not cure tinea tonsurans, though, like simple blistering, they may suffice to remove T. circinata.

Any constitutional debility, strumous condition, &c., should be treated with cod-liver oil, tonics, and good food and hygiene, which, though unable to cure the disease, by improving the general health lessen the risk of eczema, &c.

Cases of ringworm of the scalp are rarely cured within less than four to six months, and even with the most efficient and thorough treatment they may last for years. In public institutions and schools the separation of the patients and of their clothing, towels, &c., is necessary to check further spread of the disease.

TINEA VERSICOLOR—CHLOASMA—PITYRIASIS VERSICOLOR.

Definition.—A parasitic contagious disease, excited by the presence of microsporon furfur in the epidermis, usually occurring on the trunk as yellowish or pale buff-coloured patches.

Symptoms.—Tinea versicolor does not occur in childhood, and is hardly ever seen after fifty; it is met with most frequently between the ages of puberty and forty. It is far less communicable than T. circinata, and usually attacks only those who have warm, easily-perspiring skins. Occurring chiefly on the front of the chest and abdomen, on parts covered by flannel garments, it may extend to the upper arm or thigh, rarely affecting the face, scalp, or leg, and never developing on the palmar and plantar surfaces.

Small, roundish, slightly-reddened patches appear, usually symmetrically, on the trunk, extending by a slightly raised and somewhat scaly margin. The patch soon becomes pale yellow, fawn-coloured, buff, or brownish in colour; and unites with neighbouring spots, forming irregular areæ with detached roundish patches at the margin. Itching, slight or absent in most cases, may sometimes be severe, and give rise to scratching and pruritic rashes. Occasionally the hair follicles become hyperæmic, giving the patch an irregular, punctuated appearance; the pigmentary deposit may be excessive, almost sooty black, the so-called *pityriasis nigra*; or urticarial or eczematous eruptions may be excited by the parasite.

Diagnosis.—Tinea versicolor may be mistaken for a macular syphilide, or for ordinary non-parasitic chloasma (melano-derma).

The syphilide is usually accompanied by other specific eruptions, is preceded by roseola, sore throat, alopecia, &c.; does not usually itch, occurs on the trunk, face, arms, and legs indiscriminately, and is of a brownish or coppery colour. T. versicolor, though it may be met with in a syphilitic person, usually occurs *per se*; the patches frequently itch, occur most frequently on the front of the trunk, and are of a pale yellow or buff colour.

Spots of melanoderma are seen most often on exposed parts, rarely on the trunk; they are perfectly smooth, not rough or branny, and itching is not met with.

In all doubtful cases the discovery of the parasite (see morbid anatomy) on microscopic examination of the scales, will clear up the diagnosis.

Prognosis.—In those who perspire freely and do not wash the body the disease is usually chronic, and may last for years. The parasite, affecting as a rule only the superficial layers of the cuticle, can easily be got rid of by treatment.

Morbid Anatomy.—Microscopic examination of the scales scraped off from a patch of T. versicolor, and macerated in liq. potassæ, shows a network of mycelium made up of branching filaments, the segments of which are usually long and cylindrical, interspersed with roundish aggregations of large round spores, which look like bunches of grapes. The little hairs are more or less infiltrated and split up by the fungus, but the disease does not extend deeply into the epidermis or hair follicles.

Treatment.—Cleanliness, frequent washing with soft soap, and the subsequent application of sulphurous acid (1 to 4) or hyposulphite of soda lotion (℥j ad ℥j), or the inunction of a mild mercurial ointment, easily cure the disease. No internal treatment is necessary.

TINEA FAVOSA—FAVUS.

Definition.—A contagious, chronic disease, excited by the presence of acorion Schœnleinii in the epidermis, hairs, and corium; met with most frequently on the scalp.

Symptoms.—Favus, met with rarely in England, is much more common on the Continent, in Scotland, and in some parts of the United States, and, though contagious, attacks chiefly poor and dirty children. It begins on the scalp as an itching, reddish, scaly patch, resembling that of tinea tonsurans, the hairs on which are dull, but not so brittle as in ringworm. Small yellowish crusts, about the size of pins' heads, next appear round isolated hairs, which pull out more easily with their bulbs entire, not broken off; the crusts (favi), convex at first, become, as they gradually enlarge, depressed and cup-shaped in the centre, and of a bright sulphur-yellow colour. Solitary favi may enlarge till they measure ½ inch or more in diameter, or may become confluent, and by admixture with epidermis, eczematous secretions, &c., form irregular crusts. The favi have a disagreeable, mousy odour, and when removed leave a depressed pit, which is excoriated or covered with smooth epithelium. In the later stages the typical cups disappear, and the surface resembles a scaly eczema capitis. Destruction of the hair follicles and permanent alopecia are frequent results of the disease.

On the body erythematous patches or rings resembling those of T. circinata are occasionally met with; they seldom exceed ½ inch in diameter, and have not the tendency to rapid extension seen in ringworm.

It is essentially a chronic disease, lasting for many years, and, though contagious, does not seem so easily communicable as ringworm.

It is more prone to excite secondary inflammatory affections than ringworm.

In America domestic animals (cats, mice, &c.) are said frequently to transmit the disease to man.

Diagnosis.—Favus, in the early erythematous stage, resembles ringworm, but the hairs are not so brittle, are not stubbly, and pull out with their bulb entire, instead of breaking off sharply. In the developed condition the mousy-smelling, sulphur-yellow cups adherent to a hair in their centre are quite typical. In the later stages, when the cups have given way to whitish scales and flakes, or are covered over by impetiginous crusts, the discovery of the fungus under the microscope will distinguish favus from eczema in the scaly or moist and crusting stage.

Prognosis.—The disease is very chronic, and, on account of its tendency to invade the deeper tissues, resists treatment even more obstinately than ringworm of the hairy parts. Permanent alopecia is frequently caused by it, and some observers believe that it exerts a lowering influence on the general health.

Morbid Anatomy.—Microscopic examination of a portion of favus crust macerated in liq. potassæ, and subsequently tinted with iodine solution, shows a mycelium made up of ovoidal segments, averaging $\frac{1}{6000}$ inch in diameter, containing granules in their interior, and terminating in large rounded spores $\frac{1}{3500}$ inch in diameter with a distinct double contour.

Vertical sections through a favus cup show the epidermis infiltrated with spores, micrococci, and fatty granules, most numerous at the margin. In the centre of the cup the diseased hairs, which have a mycelium running longitudinally and numerous collections of spores in their substance, are met with extending down to the bulbs. Beneath them, in favi $\frac{1}{4}$ to $\frac{1}{2}$ inch in diameter, mycelial filaments are found running into the corium substance at right angles to the surface, for a more or less considerable distance ; they terminate in chaplets of spores, which, with numerous leucocytes, are found in abundance between them. The chronic exudation, and in some cases the suppuration excited by this mycelial invasion, leads to gradual wasting of the affected corium, and is perhaps the cause of the depression and loss of hair.

Treatment.—Epilation, advisable in ringworm, is here almost indispensable. The removal of crusts, blistering, and the application of the mercury and acetic acid paint, followed by hyposulphite of soda lotion or the inunction of ammonio-chloride of mercury, ung. sulph. co. (see p. 244), &c., must be persevered in for a long time. Tonics, cod-liver oil, good food, and hygiene are usually necessary.

CHAPTER XXIV.

Class B.—ERUPTIONS PRODUCED BY DRUGS.

EXTERNAL.

CERTAIN drugs, applied externally, excite eruptions of the skin.

Some, such as mustard and turpentine, cause merely a moderate hyperæmia, with but slight exudation, and are followed by branny or slight scaly desquamation and more or less lasting brown pigmentation. Others, such as croton oil, tartar emetic ointment, savin, or the juice of mezereon, excite an eczematous eruption, rapidly becoming pustular, and causing shallow ulcers, which heal, leaving whitish radiating scars, round the margin of which more or less brown pigment is usually developed. Mercurial and sulphur ointment, soda and potash soaps, also excite local eczematous eruptions.

Cantharides produces a vesicular or bullous eruption, and has been frequently used to simulate pemphigus. Arnica applied locally not unfrequently excites in the skin an erysipelatous inflammation, with considerable constitutional disturbance.

Acne, due to blocking of the sebaceous glands and their subsequent inflammation, occasionally follows the external use of tar.

INTERNAL.

Taken *internally*, belladonna or atropia, stramonium and hyoscyamus, or their active principles, cause dilatation of the pupil, dryness of the tongue and mucous membranes, delirium—often violent—muscular paresis and picking at the bed clothes, and frequently a general hyperæmic rash, most intense round the hair follicles and almost indistinguishable from the eruption of scarlatina.

Occasionally after the internal administration of quinine, or of anæsthetics, a patchy, hyperæmic, or slightly raised eruption appears on pretty large areæ of the face, neck, hands, and portions of the trunk. The patches are transitory, and it is a question whether some of them are really due to the drug or are merely erythema fugax, accidentally coinciding with its administration.

Copaiba in some cases causes a rash which at the onset resembles that of measles. Hyperæmic, slightly raised patches, at first purplish red and sometimes subsequently dark red or even hæmorrhagic in character, make their appearance on the face, trunk, and extremities. By confluence they may produce large plaques, or a diffuse paler redness may surround the individual darker papules, which arise at first round the hair follicles. More or less severe pyrexia and anorexia, with dry, brown, furred tongue and slight or severe prostration, may be met with.

Under the administration internally of arsenic, a vesicular, herpetic eruption, identical with that of zoster, sometimes developes.

Iodide of potassium or other salts of iodine taken internally produce sometimes an acneiform, but more frequently a bullous, eruption. An erythematous raised base makes its appearance, on which numerous vesicles, gradually enlarging and by confluence producing a bulla, are developed. A purpuric eruption, varying in intensity from slight petechiæ on the legs to severe P. hæmorrhagica, is also occasionally excited.

Bromide of potassium gives rise to hard tubercular swellings, resembling acne, round the sebaceous and hair follicles, which occasionally run on into pustules, or definite furuncles are produced. The cessation of the drugs, and the application of local sedatives, with purgatives internally, is usually followed by the subsidence of the eruptions.

INDEX.

LONDON : PRINTED BY
SPOTTISWOODE AND CO., NEW-STREET SQUARE
AND PARLIAMENT STREET

ATLAS OF HISTOLOGY.

By E. KLEIN, M.D., F.R.S.
AND
E. NOBLE SMITH, L.R.C.P., M.R.C.S.

A Complete Representation of the Microscopic Structure of simple and compound Tissues of Man and the higher Animals, in carefully executed Coloured Engravings, with Explanatory Text of the Figures and a concise Account of the hitherto ascertained Facts in Histology.

THE ATLAS OF HISTOLOGY

Will be completed in Twelve or Thirteen Numbers, each Number containing Three or Four royal quarto Plates and the corresponding Text.   Price 6s. each Part.

EXTRACT FROM THE AUTHOR'S PREFACE.

The work is intended to be a pictorial and literal representation of the structure of the tissues of Man and other Vertebrates; its chief aim being to teach, not so much the history of Histology, as Histology itself in its modern aspect.   The subject is divided into chapters, each receiving its separate and due share of illustrations and text.

The Illustrations are drawn and executed by Mr. E. NOBLE SMITH.   They are coloured and uncoloured.

The text comprises, besides the explanation of the illustrations themselves, a good deal of other matter that either need not be specially illustrated, being intelligible by means of the given figures, or that cannot be done so if the work is to be kept within a reasonable limit.

The subject matter will be treated in this order: First, the elementary tissues—blood, epithelium and endothelium, connective- tissues, muscular tissue, the nervous, vascular, and lymphatic system; then follows a short chapter on 'Cells in General,' after which the compound tissues will be considered *seriatim*; the alimentary canal and its glands, the respiratory organs, the urinary and genital organs, the skin and special sense organs.   The concluding chapter treats of organs the nature of which is not sufficiently well known, as the suprarenal capsule, the thyroid and coccygeal gland.

London: SMITH, ELDER, & CO., 15 Waterloo Place.
U

SMITH, ELDER, & CO.'S PUBLICATIONS.

COMPENDIUM of HISTOLOGY. Twenty-four Lectures. By HEINRICH FREY, Professor. Translated from the German, by permission of the Author, by GEORGE R. CUTTER, M.D. With 208 Illustrations. 8vo. 12s.

ELEMENTS of HUMAN PHYSIOLOGY. By Dr. L. HERMANN, Professor of Physiology in the University of Zurich. Second Edition. Entirely recast from the Sixth German Edition, with very copious Additions and many additional Woodcuts. By ARTHUR GAMGEE, M.D., F.R.S., Brackenbury Professor of Physiology in Owens College, Manchester, and Examiner in Physiology in the University of Edinburgh. Second Edition. Demy 8vo. 16s.

SURGERY: its PRINCIPLES and PRACTICE. By TIMOTHY HOLMES, F.R.C.S., Surgeon to St. George's Hospital. With upwards of 400 Illustrations. Second Edition. Royal 8vo. 30s.

The ESSENTIALS of BANDAGING; including the Management of Fractures and Dislocations, with Directions for using other Surgical Apparatus. With 128 Engravings. By BERKELEY HILL, M.B. Lond., F.R.C.S. Third Edition, Revised and Enlarged. Fcp. 8vo. 4s. 6d.

The STUDENT'S MANUAL of VENEREAL DISEASES. Being a concise Description of those Affections and of their Treatment. By BERKELEY HILL, M.B., Professor of Clinical Surgery in University College, London; Surgeon to the University College, and Surgeon to the Lock Hospital; and by ARTHUR COOPER, late House Surgeon to the Lock Hospital. Post 8vo. 2s. 6d.

A HANDBOOK of OPHTHALMIC SURGERY. By BENJAMIN THOMPSON LOWNE, F.R.C.S., Ophthalmic Surgeon to the Great Northern Hospital. Crown 8vo. 6s.

A TREATISE on the THEORY and PRACTICE of MEDICINE. By JOHN SYER BRISTOWE, M.D. Lond., F.R.C.P., Physician to St. Thomas's Hospital; Joint Lecturer in Medicine to the Royal College of Surgeons; formerly Examiner in Medicine to the University of London; and Lecturer on General Pathology and on Physiology at St. Thomas's Hospital. Second Edition. 8vo. 21s.

London: SMITH, ELDER, & CO., 15 Waterloo Place.

SMITH, ELDER, & CO.'S PUBLICATIONS.

CLINICAL MANUAL for the STUDY of MEDICAL CASES. Edited by JAMES FINLAYSON, M.D., Physician and Lecturer on Clinical Medicine in the Glasgow Western Infirmary, &c. With Special Chapters by Professor GAIRDNER on the Physiognomy of Disease; Professor STEPHENSON on Disorders of the Female Organs; Dr. ALEXANDER ROBERTSON on Insanity; Dr. SAMSON GEMMEL on Physical Diagnosis; Mr. JOSEPH COATS on Laryngoscopy, and also on the Method of performing *Post-mortem* Examinations. Crown 8vo., with numerous Illustrations, 12s. 6d.

An INTRODUCTION to the STUDY of CLINICAL MEDICINE: being a Guide to the Investigation of Disease, for the Use of Students. By OCTAVIUS STURGES, M.D. (Cantab.), F.R.C.P., Physician to Westminster Hospital. Crown 8vo. 4s. 6d.

AUSCULTATION and PERCUSSION, together with the other Methods of Physical Examination of the Chest. By SAMUEL GEE, M.D. With Illustrations. New Edition. Fcp. 8vo. 6s.

The NOTATION CASE BOOK. Designed by HENRY VEALE, M.D., Assistant-Professor of Military Medicine in the Army Medical School; Surgeon-Major, Army Medical Department, &c. Oblong crown 8vo. for the Pocket, 6s.

A TREATISE on the SCIENCE and PRACTICE of MID-WIFERY. By W. S. PLAYFAIR, M.D., F.R.C.P., Professor of Obstetric Medicine in King's College; Physician for the Diseases of Women and Children to King's College Hospital; Examiner in Midwifery to the University of London, and lately to the Royal College of Physicians; Vice-President to the Obstetrical Society, &c. Second Edition. 2 vols. demy 8vo. with 166 Illustrations, 28s.

A MANUAL of MIDWIFERY for MIDWIVES. By FANCOURT BARNES, M.D. Aber., M.R.C.P. Lond., Physician to the General Lying-in Hospital; Assistant-Physician to the Royal Maternity Charity of London; Physician for the Diseases of Women to the St. George's and St. James's Dispensary. Crown 8vo. with numerous Illustrations, price 6s.

NOTES of DEMONSTRATIONS of PHYSIOLOGICAL CHE-MISTRY. By S. W. MOORE, Junior Demonstrator of Practical Physiology at St. George's Medical School, Fellow of the Chemical Society, &c. Crown 8vo. 3s. 6d.

London: SMITH, ELDER, & CO., 15 Waterloo Place.